become a
Wellness
Champion

become a
Wellness
Champion

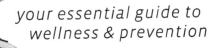

*your essential guide to
wellness & prevention*

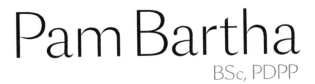

Pam Bartha
BSc, PDPP

Wellness Publishing International
Kelowna, B.C., 2011

FIRST EDITION

Published by Wellness Publishing International

Illustrations	David Fletcher: www.krop.com/davidfletcher
Cover & Text design	Puckett: www.puckett.com
Cover photos	Timothy Geiss / Shutterstock (*pill bottle*)
	Sari ONeal / Shutterstock (*butterfly*)
Editing	Unger & Knight: www.ungerandknight.com
	Matt Smartt: www.puckett.com

Library and Archives Canada Cataloguing in Publication

Bartha, Pam
    Become a wellness champion : your essential guide to wellness & prevention / Pam Bartha.

Includes index.
Issued also in an electronic format.
ISBN 978-0-9869267-0-9

    1. Health. 2. Well-being. 3. Medicine, Preventive. I. Title.

RA776.B27 2011   613   C2011-905450-7

This book is dedicated with much love
to Kevin, my soul mate.

Pam Bartha

CONTENTS

SECTION TWO: THE FOUR PILLARS OF WELLNESS

FOREWORD

A NOTE FROM DR. FRED PESCATORE

Becoming a Wellness Champion doesn't require much. In fact it merely requires one thing—determination. Most people don't think of their health as something that needs attention every day, yet in fact it needs attention multiple times throughout the day. Our health is something that is so important that it must take priority, or we can choose to sit back and wonder "How did I put on so much weight?" "How could I have become a diabetic?" "Why did I get cancer?"

The reason health takes so much attention is because health begins with what we eat, how much we sleep, how stressed we are and even if we are in a relationship or not. Each and every one of those factors and many others can make us healthy or not. The choices we make and the decisions we make affect our health on a—dare I say it—hourly basis. The positive decisions for health can be made but you need determination to do so on a consistent basis.

You also need a book like, *Becoming a Wellness Champion*. There is so much confusing health and wellness information available through so many sources it has become impossible to cipher through it. We are bombarded with what is and isn't healthy, and quite often what is demonized today is deified tomorrow—so what do you do? You consult a source. You look for someone without an agenda and you look for someone you can trust and that is, Pam Bartha.

She has her own compelling story and believe me, there are many more like her out there. She has the courage to tell her story in a public forum. There is no better advocate for health and wellness than someone who has been there; someone who has literally taken one for the team and has defied all odds. These are the people who have no agenda other than to share their school-of-hard-knocks knowledge with the world.

Pam lays it out well when she discusses the agenda that is big health care. The industry is not there to make any of us well, but rather to get us dependent on pharmaceutical medications from as young an age as possible and to make us unhealthy by poisoning our food supply.

This is why it is critical to have the same determination for health and wellness that you have for anything else in your life, and that includes your career, children, spouse, etc. Health is the most important thing you can have and you will never realize it until you don't have it.

So the only way to have it is: practice, practice, practice. It is a conversation you need to have in your mind every day. Whenever you are deciding what to eat, whether to go to the gym or not, or even staying up late to watch a movie. Each of these simple decisions will affect your health. Just choose the right ones. Start somewhere and honestly be committed to this as if your life depends on it—because quite frankly, it does.

Our health care system is perfect for catastrophic illness, but not for prevention. You have to be your own advocate for being healthy and *Become a Wellness Champion* is a great place to start that journey. I hope you enjoy reading the book as much as I did.

FRED PESCATORE, MD, MPH, CCN
www.drpescatore.com

Dr. Fred Pescatore is an internationally recognized health, nutrition and weight loss expert. He is author of the *New York Times* best-selling book *The Hamptons Diet*, and the number one best-selling children's health book *Feed Your Kids Well*, among many other titles.

A NOTE FROM DR. CAROLYN DEAN

Become a Wellness Champion is a call to action from a courageous and powerful woman. Pam Bartha's power comes from taking responsibility for her own health. One of her finest statements is— "Your health is your responsibility. You cannot afford to leave it in the hands of any expert!"

Pam learned that specialists are only knowledgeable about their own field and they certainly didn't know everything about her body.

In 1988, at age 28, Pam was diagnosed with multiple sclerosis. She was told by her neurologist that it was only a matter of time before she would become completely disabled. Unfortunately this doctor was playing god. He was adamant that there was nothing that she could do to change the prognosis of her disease. He even warned her against snake oil cures, saying they were useless.

She then made the conscious decision to be personally responsible for her health and began researching for ways to achieve optimal health. Over the years she's tried many safe therapies and natural supplements. She discovered that when she treated silent infections in her body, namely yeast overgrowth, her health began to improve. It was like a scientific experiment with only one person in the study. She found that some things helped and others did not as she learned and grew in her experience. Now, twenty years later she is still drug-free and symptom-free!

That's what makes *Become a Wellness Champion* such an important book. Because if Pam can do it, so can you!

Beyond her amazing story of recovery, Pam challenges the reader to become a Wellness Champion and has been inspiring others to take charge of their own health for many years. She provides four pillars of wellness to show you how to accomplish this. In my experience it boils down to a willingness to accept responsibility for what you have been eating, drinking, smoking and thinking.

Another aspect of the book I like is the scientific validation for her work. This comes from the high school science teacher part of Pam. *Become a Wellness Champion* is not just a personal story of her quest but a book that you can show your doctor to gain support for your own journey.

I hope you are as inspired by Pam's book as I am. Within its pages is the future of medicine which necessarily must come from outside the medical/pharmaceutical industry.

DR. CAROLYN DEAN, MD, ND
http://drcarolyndean.com/

Dr. Dean is a medical doctor and naturopathic doctor. She has been in the forefront of the natural medicine revolution for more than 30 years. She is the author/co-author of 22 health and wellness books.

ABOUT THE AUTHOR

I am a wellness researcher, educator and coach. My personal story is powerful and I have coached many people whom I call Wellness Champions. These courageous folks have taken charge of their health and have each improved their quality of life radically. I have a Bachelor of Science degree, and have studied integrative health since 1988. I am excited to share my story and insights with you because I am passionate about empowering others to improve their quality of life.

Years ago, I suffered a serious health challenge and I know how scary and devastating poor health can be. At the age of 28, I was diagnosed with multiple sclerosis (MS). I had always considered myself an active, healthy person and was shocked to be informed that I had a degenerative disease. It is amazing how quickly and how dramatically your life can change overnight.

It is important to share with you that at the time I was diagnosed, I was a healthy young mother. I ate a healthy diet (healthier than most), was at my ideal weight and I was active. I asked myself, "How could this happen to me?" I share this story because many of you ask the same question: "Why are so many seemingly healthy people becoming so sick?"

I was diagnosed with MS at a university MS clinic in June of 1988. The neurologist told me that it was only a matter of time before I would become completely disabled, and he was adamant that there was nothing that I could do to change the prognosis of the disease. He said that people would tell me about all kinds of snake oil cures, but he assured me that there was nothing that would cure the disease that I had. I left the clinic feeling devastated and that my life was over. All that I could think about was that I would be a burden to my husband, and would not be able to care for my two young children.

I experienced extreme fatigue, headaches, weakness and tingling in my legs as well as a severe case of optic neuritis. The optic neuritis was so strong that I lost all vision in my left eye. It was as if I had a black patch over my left eye for several weeks. I was a mess physically and emotionally. My mom stepped in to help as I could no longer care for my young family, let alone myself.

I was clueless as to what science and medicine didn't know. I expected to be fixed by the experts, but soon realized that there was little that they could do to help me. MS was a mysterious *thing* taking over my body. The cause for MS was and still is unknown, and no one could tell me how quickly or slowly the disease would progress. I knew that MS was a serious disease but I had no idea how debilitating it could be. The diagnosis of MS provided a name for the symptoms I was experiencing, which would help the neurologist determine which drug to prescribe. I was informed that the drug wouldn't fix me, but might slow down the progression of the disease. *Might* was the operative word.

Shortly thereafter, my mother-in-law gave me the book *The Yeast Connection*, by Dr. William Crook. In the late 1980s the wellness revolution had not yet started. I had never been introduced to the notion of complimentary or integrative health. I was also not familiar with Candida or yeast as I had never experienced yeast infections in the past... or so I thought. As I read *The Yeast Connection*, I could relate to many of the symptoms in the survey. I was fascinated and excited about the possibility that there was hope that I could improve my quality of life.

This opened a new world of possibilities for me and was a major turning point in my life. I made the decision to be proactive with my health and began researching globally for ways to achieve optimal wellness. Over the years I have tried many safe therapies and natural supplements: some things helped and others did not. No matter how frustrated I was at times, I always believed that my journey would serve some purpose and that some good would come from it. I am very grateful that I have been and am able to enjoy an active and healthy life for more than 20 years now, without the use of pharmaceuticals.

By taking responsibility for my health and building the Four Pillars of Wellness, I have been able to complete a Bachelor of Science degree, become a certified teacher and have my third child. I have been blessed to coach hundreds of others over the past ten years and play a small part in each of their successes. I enjoy an active lifestyle, which includes horse riding, biking, skiing, camping and traveling.

Once again, I would like to state that the knowledge in this book is designed for educational purposes and is not intended to replace the necessary measures of a health care professional. It is not intended to cure, treat, or mitigate any health condition or disease. I am a wellness coach, educator and researcher, not a health care professional. I have a unique perspective in that I have walked the walk with disease, have an extensive science and nutrition background, and have coached hundreds of people in wellness. I have valuable insights that I want to share with you—insights that are not readily understood or accepted by our traditional medical model; insights that I have learned personally, the hard way.

I was given a second chance to enjoy an excellent quality of life and I am passionate about helping you achieve optimal health as well. From personal experience, I do believe that if you are committed to improving your health, you can also improve your quality of life enormously. The choice is really up to you. Wellness is a continuum, and for the most part you get to choose the level of wellness you want to experience. If your health challenges are great, you may have to work a bit harder and be diligent, but the end result is so worth it. Regardless of your diagnoses or which health club you belong to, you can choose to live a healthier life.

HOW THIS BOOK IS LAID OUT

Section One takes an honest look at the present state of health care: its philosophy, its limitations, as well as the major health issues we are facing as a society. It is important to understand where we are, how we reached this point, and the global nature of these issues before we can even consider moving forward.

The second section of the book will outline the solution, namely, the Four Pillars of Wellness. This will be your simple, lifelong blueprint for success in wellness. The success that I have enjoyed over the past twenty-some years is the result of building my Four Pillars of Wellness and the same is true for many others.

The third section will focus on women's health issues while the fourth section will challenge men and women to become Wellness Champions using principles from the Four Pillars of Wellness. Wellness Champions not only value quality of life for themselves, but also care about the well-being of others around them. Although this section is found at the end of the book, it may in fact be the start of a new journey. Thus I invite you to join me on the road to becoming a Wellness Champion.

I have provided peer-reviewed research for the skeptics and for those who wish to investigate these topics further. The many sources used to produce this book can be found in the Reference Section at the back.

The reality is that you must take responsibility for your health and this book will help you to do just that. If you implement the information I've gathered here from the knowledge of the experts and from my journey through illness, I believe that your quality of life will improve immensely.

PREFACE

ealth care is big business, and with many stakeholders carving out their share of the market a thick smoke screen has developed, clouding our understanding of wellness. We live in a developed country that offers the most advanced medical care in the world, yet disease trends and health care costs continue to rise. Many of us are finally waking up to the realization that our health care system is not living up to its promise and that the conventional medical model has, in many cases, profound limitations.

As we search for solutions outside this system, we are confronted with thousands of supplements and therapies. Companies offer expensive newfangled products and therapies that are touted as the answer to all our woes. We desperately try one complementary alternative treatment after the next, spending hundreds or thousands of dollars, often with limited success. Most of us are confused, frustrated and desperately searching for an answer.

This book will clear the smoke screen overshadowing our present concept of wellness. My goal is to simplify wellness for you. I do not have all the answers. But the knowledge and insights that I have gained over the years have the potential to improve your quality of life profoundly. It has for myself and many others.

This book will challenge many of your fundamental beliefs around health and sickness. Many of you are ready for this message and will run with it, while some will remain skeptical, resistant and stuck. Even so, a seed will be planted and as you hear this message over and over again from other sources in the coming years, my hope is that you will eventually embrace this new way of thinking about health and wellness for the sake of both you and your family. It is ironic that this philosophy is not really new at all. Our health care has become so high-tech that we have forgotten even the most basic principles that were well understood by our forebearers.

Much of the information that I will share in this book is based on simple principles that will make sense to you. You will ask yourself, "could it really be that simple?" My answer is yes, it is that simple.

But unfortunately, simple does not support exorbitant profits. So many unrelated mysterious diseases have been created which require unique costly pharmaceuticals and medical treatments.

This book is a resource that will provide you with insights and an understanding of wellness that will better equip you to take responsibility for your health and improve your interaction with health care providers where and when it is necessary. If you are healthy, use these insights to stay well and share them with others you care about. Enjoy wellness and pay it forward. Your health is your responsibility. You cannot afford to leave it solely in the hands of any one expert!

Where We Are and How We Got Here

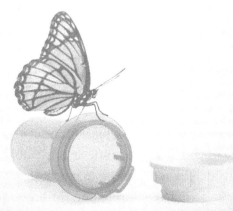

1 Which Health Club Do You Currently Belong To?

THE HYPOCHONDRIACS

Are you at your wits end with respect to your health? There are specific requirements to be included in this exclusive club. You have seen countless specialists (or so you thought) and had all the tests done only to be informed that you are perfectly healthy. You know that something is wrong with your health but no one can tell you what it is.

You've spent a fortune trying complementary therapies but have experienced little improvement to your health. You suspect that certain foods might make your symptoms worse and you are not sure what you should eat. In fact, it would actually be easier if you didn't have to eat.

Your doctor may have informed you not to come back because he/she cannot help you. Or, maybe you have been told that it's all in your head. Even if you haven't formally been labelled a hypochondriac, you feel that others may wind up thinking this about you if you keep complaining, so instead you hide your suffering. In public you pretend that all is well, but inside you feel miserable much of the time. No one can possibly understand what you are going through. Your dire physical state is on your mind all the time and you would like a break from it all. You say to yourself, "Why can't I just be normal like everyone else…to be able to eat normal foods and just live without this constant concern about my health?" You are left feeling hopeless and depressed.

THE NOT-SO-RELIEVED DIAGNOSED

To be part of this group, you're fortunate enough to have a diagnosis; you actually have a label for the symptoms that you suffer with. At first you are relieved (but not happy) to receive this diagnosis. With it you assumed the specialists could fix you, but you quickly discovered that there is no known cause or cure for your demise, I mean disease.

The good news is that this label will add credibility to your complaints and will also help the specialists determine which pharmaceuticals you need. You are told that you now have a permanent health condition that you must live with for the rest of your life. Furthermore, the financial cost and side effects of the drugs are downright depressing. As a result, your doctor will probably have to add antidepressants to your drug protocol. And to top all of this, you are informed that in time you may need to include other medications to help you deal with the long-term side effects of the pharmaceuticals that you are currently taking to control the original problem. How did this happen to you anyway? You were such a healthy person.

THE DELUSIONALLY HEALTHY

You can only be part of this group if you know that you are healthy. How do you know this? Well, because you've been told this by your doctor and you don't have any major diseases—not like The Diagnosed group. You were fortunate to be born healthy and you are confident that you will remain healthy because you have a strong constitution. A little voice inside assures you will be healthy forever. Sure, you may have minor nuisances such as weight gain, allergies, insomnia, joint stiffness, high blood pressure or possibly high cholesterol, but that's completely normal, right?

Your job is stressful and takes up much of your time so you really don't have the time to prepare healthy meals or exercise regularly. You do your best and try to eat right, but you are on the run most of the time. Getting enough sleep is a major challenge: let's face it, it just doesn't happen regularly. Sure, your life might be a bit out of balance, but you seem to be coping just fine.

CHAMPIONS FOR WELLNESS

The majority of people who become members of this club were originally members of one of the first three clubs. Most of you have been there and done that with sickness. Suffering with poor health motivated you to search out answers and change your lifestyle. A smaller percentage of you joined this exclusive club because you watched someone close to you go through the pain and agony of sickness and you decided that this was not the road you wanted to take.

As a Wellness Champion you decided to take responsibility for your health and be proactive in doing it. Adopting a healthy lifestyle was the only option that you would consider. You understand that well-

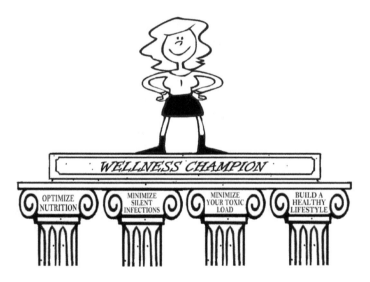

ness is not a God-given right; it is something that must be earned by following basic fundamental principles. You realize that sickness is a costly venture and you are aware that our current health care model is unsustainable, so you work hard at minimizing your dependence upon the system. Quality of life is far more important to you than satisfying a sweet tooth or other unhealthy craving, and without optimal health, you won't be able to do the things you love to do. You enjoy a very active life but balance is something that you are constantly aware of and strive for. You are purpose-driven and share this message of hope with others who are searching for answers. You are a true champion!

> **Which club do you currently belong to?**
> **Which club will you choose?**

HOW DO I KNOW THESE CLUBS SO WELL?

I have been a member of each club at some point in my life. I have also coached many others who have worked their way out of the first three groups to become Wellness Champions. No matter which group you belong to at this time, be assured that only you can change the course of your future.

I believe that you can improve your quality of life immensely. It will require that you evaluate your beliefs around wellness, learn and implement new strategies that really work, and adopt a new wellness philosophy. If this is your desire, let's get started!

2 Knowledge is Not Always Power

WELLNESS AND OUR BELIEFS

The new buzz word is wellness. In fact, we are embarking on a wellness revolution. Many of us are dissatisfied with our quality of health and we are searching for answers. We are sick and tired of being sick and tired, and we are looking for ways to improve our quality of life. We are also becoming aware that our health care system will not financially sustain the burden of our flawed *sickness care* philosophy and our poor lifestyle choices; it is expensive and many of us would like to minimize our dependence upon it.

Wellness occurs on a continuum, or scale. It is dynamic and always changing, because things are constantly changing in our lives. Our levels of stress, physical activity, exposure to sunshine and bad microbes, what we eat, and the hours of sleep we get change day by day.

RATING YOURSELF ON THE WELLNESS SCALE

Let's say that wellness is rated on a scale of 0–10, where zero means that you are basically dead and 10 means that you experience perfect wellness. A perfect score of 10 may be difficult if not impossible to reach because we cannot avoid the continued assaults from our environment. I believe that most of us can attain close to a ten if we choose, but it will definitely be more challenging to reach this goal if we suffer from poor health. From personal experience I believe that most of us should be able to enjoy optimal health and reach a score of at least 7 or higher.

If this is the case, then why aren't we all fit and healthy? We live in a land of plenty and are bombarded with information about health from the media, the Internet, magazines and books. Yet obesity is epidemic, disease trends are on the rise and health care systems are unsustainable. Much of the information we receive is confusing, contradictory and often inaccurate. Magic pills and special diets promise a quick fix but in time we realize there is no quick fix. Is more information and education the answer? I am not convinced.

GROOMING HEALTHY WELLNESS BELIEFS

Being informed is important, but there is definitely more to this issue if we are to be properly empowered. I believe we must first look at our core beliefs around health. We may think that we are making our decisions based on facts, but in reality our beliefs are making decisions for us all the time. This may sound a bit *out there* or new to some of you, but bear with me as I explain.

The majority of our personal beliefs about wellness were established when we were young. Some of our beliefs serve us well but others actually stop us from succeeding in life. In his book, *If How-to's Were Enough, We Would All Be Skinny, Rich and Happy*, Brian Klemmer explains that if we want to create big change in our lives in a short period of time, we must begin by looking at our beliefs about health and wellness.

Do we believe that there is no hope because we have been told this by an *expert*? Do we believe that our genetics prevent us from achieving a perfect body shape? Do we believe that we inherited a bad heart? Do we believe that we don't have time to exercise, or that healthy foods are expensive? This *beliefs* list is endless and it keeps us stuck in old, ineffective ways of thinking.

It is really important to explore and determine all the beliefs that you hold around health and wellness, then list the benefits and costs of each belief. What are sickness, obesity, and other related health conditions costing you both financially and with respect to your quality of life? Answering these questions will help you see which beliefs may actually be stopping you from living the life you desire.

For meaningful change to occur in our life, our intention (or determination to carry out our goal) and the reasons why we want to accomplish our goal must be crystal clear and strong. What do you want to accomplish and why? Why must you succeed? How committed are you to your intention? If your intention is not rock solid, you probably won't follow through. You must have a bigger reason (or *why*) to make significant change than the short term inconvenience or pain that comes with change. Why do you want to live at your ideal body weight or change your lifestyle? What will the benefits be if you do make the change and what price will you pay if you don't commit to improving your health? What's at stake? You must be honest with yourself and consider the long-term consequences of your actions. The more real this is for you, the stronger your intention will be to change and the more likely you will succeed. Take a few minutes to complete the following activities. Use extra paper if more space is required.

MY INTENTION AND MY "WHY"

What do I Intend to accomplish?

○

Why must I succeed? What will my life look like when I accomplish my goal? How will I feel? Make this section as detailed as possible.

○

○

○

○

MY WELLNESS BELIEFS

My Wellness Belief	What are the benefits of holding onto this belief?	What price will I pay for holding onto this belief?
Belief #1		
Belief #2		
Belief #3		

My intention of getting well was extremely strong because if I didn't follow through, change my lifestyle and seek out solutions, I would have become totally disabled. This made it much easier for me to say *no* to a piece of cheesecake or a glass of wine while out with my friends. Eating junk food while I was trying to regain my health wasn't an option. My desire to live a quality life (which was my *why*) was much greater than the short-term satisfaction (or benefit) that I received from eating unhealthy food.

It is critical that we as parents groom constructive wellness beliefs and habits in our children. When our children experience the benefits of being physically fit, having lots of energy, and feeling and looking great at a young age they will value this throughout their lives. The biggest impact on the health of our children comes from family and life at home. I understand how challenging it is to raise children. Many families are struggling to make ends meet. Nonetheless, the cost of ignoring this is far too great. Parents must look at their beliefs about health and wellness and decide if their beliefs are serving or costing their family. As we raise children who value and choose optimal health we will begin to see a change in our health care system. Wellness is a lifestyle, a way of life; it isn't a quick fix.

If your desire to create change in your life is deep, and your why is clear and strong, it is helpful to share this with someone you trust—someone who will support and encourage you, someone who will hold you accountable until you achieve your success.

For the most part, the level of wellness that we experience today is the direct product of the beliefs that we hold. Any valuable knowledge that you obtain from this book will only benefit you if your beliefs around wellness will allow it. Remember that the level of wellness you experience is your responsibility.

3 The State of Health Care: It's Not Working

Before we move forward, it is important to understand where we're at with respect to health care and how we got here and to evaluate how well this is working for us. As we understand the dynamics, values and philosophies of the various industries that are involved in our health, we will be better equipped to make sure that our success is not temporary, but that it lasts a lifetime.

Let's start by examining the system that supports and promotes our health.

INCREASED HEALTH CARE SPENDING—A GLOBAL CRISIS

In many countries around the world, government spending on health care has been growing faster on average than government revenue. Health care spending has been rising faster than economic growth in all of the Organization for Economic Co-operation and Development (OECD) countries.[1] In these countries, the average ratio of health spending to gross domestic product (GDP) has grown from 7.8% in 2000 to 9.0% in 2008.[2]

In 2006, IBM Global Services, a division of the IBM Institute for Business Value, published a report called Health Care 2015: Win-Win or Lose-Lose. This report states that health care is currently in a state of crisis and the authors conclude that if current trends continue and change is not made, many health care systems around the world will become unsustainable by the year 2015.[3]

The marked increase in health care spending is the result of increased pharmaceutical costs,[4] new technologies and procedures, and an aging population.[5] If health care spending continues to grow faster than the economy, existing taxes will likely be increased, new taxes may be introduced and/or health care spending will be reduced, resulting in longer wait times and fewer funded services. Take a look at the daunting trends.

Canada

The Fraser Institute of Health reported that during the period from 1997/98–2007/08, health care spending in Canada grew at an unsustainable pace in nine of the ten provinces.[6] They warn that this alarming trend does not take into account the aging baby boomer population that will further burden the health care system and bring this crisis to a head much sooner than predicted.

In Ontario, health care spending is predicted to account for two thirds of the provincial government budget by 2017, and 100% by 2026.[7]

In September 2006, the government of British Columbia launched Conversation on Health, the largest and most wide-ranging public discussion the province has conducted on health and our health care system. In their publication, *Join the Conversation on Health*, they stated that growing health care costs in B.C. are unsustainable and they predict that B.C.'s health care spending could account for more than 70% of the total provincial budget by the year 2017.[8]

United States

Health care spending in the U.S. has consistently grown faster than the economy since the 1960s. The U.S. spent $2 trillion on health care in 2005 and is expected to spend $4 trillion in 2015. According to the OECD, the U.S. spent more than twice as much on health care per person in 2008 than any other OECD country,[9] yet the World Health Organization ranked the U.S. 37th in overall health care performance, and the OECD ranked the U.S. 22nd in life expectancy among the 30 OECD countries.[10]

China

Despite economic and social successes over the past 25 years, 29% of China's rural population and 36% of its urban population cannot afford medical treatment.[11]

SICKNESS CARE: A FLAWED PHILOSOPHY

Our system of health care is really more accurately described by the term *sickness care*. For the most part, we access the system when our health is suffering. I believe that more of our health care budget should be spent on prevention education. OECD countries spend on average only 3% of their health care budgets on prevention and public awareness programs.[12] Sickness care is expensive and does not promote wellness.

If health care systems are not sustainable, why aren't governments dealing with this problem? While we occasionally hear about the state of health care in the news, this dilemma continues to grow. Is it wise to pour additional tax dollars into a system that is unsustainable? I don't think so. I believe that it is not being dealt with because of the strong resistance that governments would face if they made the necessary changes. There are three groups that would offer the most resistance because they have a vested interest in maintaining the status quo.

RESISTANCE FROM THE BIG THREE

a. Our resistance

Canadians have become accustomed to an almost free health care system. We either have an extended medical plan through work, or make monthly payments for Medicare, which do not reflect the true cost of the services we use or the treatments we receive. As of January 2011, in British Columbia for example, a single person pays $726 annually for Medicare while a family of 3 or more pays $1308 annually.[13] In Alberta, the government no longer collects premiums for basic Medicare as of 2010.[14] Ontario collects minimal premiums depending on the person's taxable income.[15] In B.C. and Ontario, students or low income families can apply for premium assistance and, depending on their circumstance, are able to receive up to 100% assistance.

Most of us have no idea what true costs are associated with using our health care system. Table 1 will help us to appreciate the true costs of several common acute care treatments in Canada. Acute care hospital stays refer to short term surgical and medical treatments given to people who have unexpected medical issues and need immediate assessment and treatment.

Table 1. The average unit cost of acute care hospital stays by medical condition in Canada 2004-2005—Cost attributed to the treatment of primary diagnosis and complexities [16]

Medical Condition	Avg. Unit Cost ($)
Forearm fracture	$5000
Lower leg or ankle fracture	$5800
Pneumonia	$7000
Heart disease	$10,000
Atrial Fibrillation	$24,000
Diabetes	$10,000
Asthma	$2700
Multiple sclerosis	$10,000
Crohn's disease & ulcerative colitis	$9000
Alzheimer's	$18,000
Dementia	$17,000
Malignant neoplasm	$10,000

The unit costs in Table 1 are averages. Actual costs do vary from province to province yet these staggering figures show us that the true cost of health care far exceeds revenue generated by Medicare premiums.

The following is a list of average general practitioner (GP) fees (depending on age of the patient) in British Columbia:[17]

- A visit—$38
- A complete exam—$85

Americans paid approximately $100 on average to primary care physicians which includes general practice, family medicine, internal medicine and pediatric physicians. In the U.S., citizens paid on average approximately one-fifth of the total expenses for their visits to primary care physicians out of their own pocket. The balance was paid by private insurance and Medicare.[18]

> Most of us have no idea what true costs are associated with using our health care system.

The Canadian and American physician fees that are listed do not include the fees of medical specialists which are considerably higher.

A heavily subsidized Canadian health care system is all that we have known and we believe that we are entitled to it, after-all we pay our taxes. Whenever we feel the need to visit a doctor we just make an appointment or drop in to a walk-in clinic. We abuse our health, find ourselves sick, run to the doctor and then expect our doctor to prescribe a medication that will fix us so that we can carry on. In Canada, we are able to see the doctor as often as we want and for whatever we want. Now that the U.S. government has allowed pharmaceutical companies to advertise their drugs in American advertisements, we can even inform our doctor which drug we want.

This system does not penalize us for choosing an unhealthy, inactive lifestyle. We are able to smoke, live a sedentary lifestyle, regularly indulge in processed foods and alcohol and use the system as often as we want with no consequence.

We like this system because it is relatively easy to access and doesn't hold us accountable for our poor choices. We foolishly believe that government revenue is able to support the financial burden of our unhealthy lifestyle—yet the reality is that the system is not sustainable, and therefore we must take responsibility for our health and minimize our dependence on the health care system.

b. The medical community's resistance

I believe that the vast majority of doctors chose their profession because they really want to make a difference in the lives of others. They made a considerable investment in both time and finances to become a medical doctor. The problem lies in the philosophy of the training they received in medical school and the influence of pharmaceutical companies during that training. The conventional medical model's philosophy is more aptly termed disease management through the use of pharmaceuticals and medical procedures. Traditionally, medical schools have not valued prevention and integrative health.

The pharmaceutical industry's influence on medical students and doctors has gained much attention in the past few years. In 2005, a national U.S. survey conducted on 1,143 third-year medical students reported that on average the students were exposed to one gift or one sponsored activity from a pharmaceutical company each week. Over 80% of the students believed that they were entitled to these gifts. The study concluded that as a group these medical students were at risk for unrecognized influence by the marketing efforts of the drug companies.[19]

This influence continues as medical students become physicians. Drug companies market directly to patients through advertising, and to physicians through gifts, free samples, continuing medical education, and detailing (educating doctors about the drug). Researchers from the University of California reported that doctors spend more hours receiving continuing education from pharmaceutical supported courses than from medical schools or professional societies.[20] In 2004, researchers estimated that the U.S. pharmaceutical industry spent $57 billion on promotional advertising, and of this figure approximately

$61,000 was spent on promotion that year per physician.[21]

The Canadian medical community is not immune to the influence of the pharmaceutical industry either. The pharmaceutical companies spend an estimated $1.7 billion each year marketing their products to Canadian physicians.[22] Dr. Joel Lexchin, a physician of the emergency department of Toronto hospital, says that freebies from pharmaceutical companies are still common.[23]

A study published in the *McGill Journal of Medicine* found that medical students at the University of Western Ontario, Canada were "generally not opposed to interacting with and receiving gifts from the pharmaceutical industry."[24]

In Canada between the years 2000–2004 approximately 70% of continuing education programs accredited by the College of Family Physicians of Canada had some pharmaceutical funding.[25] In addition, between the years 2003–2004 pharmaceutical companies spent approximately $340 million on meetings in Canada. Wayne Kondro reveals alarming news in a 2008 *Canadian Medical Association Journal* article. He states that Irving Gold, vice president of the Association of Faculties of Medicine of Canada, Government Relations and External Affairs says:

> ...no national guidelines or overarching policy framework exists in Canada comparable to that proposed for the U.S. Individual Canadian medical faculties have their own policies and there is widespread variation across the country in terms of attitudes and policies towards industry handouts, Gold says. No effort has been made to compile a compendium of policies existing within Canadian schools, nor an effort made to develop a national policy framework or guidelines.[27]

The conventional medical model has had the luxury of monopolizing the health care market in North America for many years. Most of our health care funds are allocated to the medical system. It is evident that a more preventative integrative approach to health care would be more effective and feasible, yet the medical system is resistant to give up this control.

c. Big Pharma's resistance

In Canada, pharmaceutical spending has risen faster than all other health care spending. Drug spending has more than doubled from 1991 to 2001.[28] This trend is true for the United States also.

Pharmaceutical spending in the U.S. has increased almost six-fold since 1990, from $40.3 billion to $234.1 billion in 2008.[29] Excessive spending is a global dilemma. The OECD reported that growth in pharmaceutical spending from 1997 to 2005 had outstripped growth in total health spending in most OECD countries.[30]

Increased drug spending is the result of more people using drugs and newer, more expensive drugs coming onto the market.[31]

If more people are using drugs then we must be getting healthier...right?

Not so! Even though the U.S. spends more on health care than any other country, the World Health Organization ranked the U.S. 72nd out of 191 countries on overall level of health of the population, while Canada ranked 35th.[32] These rankings are not impressive considering what we spend on health care.

Before I continue, I would like to clarify that I am not against the use of pharmaceuticals. There are times when they are necessary and save lives. I believe that the use of pharmaceuticals today is excessive. Let's examine why this is so.

Pharmaceutical companies are corporations. Their mandate is to make money, not to cure people. In fact "pharmaceutical manufacturing was the most profitable industry in the U.S. from 1995–2002, and in 2008 it ranked third with profits (after taxes) of about 19 percent."[33]

Drug companies are in business to patent products that will provide their shareholders with the best return on investment. For us to expect anything else is foolish.

Some people still believe that drug companies charge high prices for their drugs because they have invested so heavily in research. Researchers at York University estimate that the U.S. pharmaceutical industry spends almost twice as much on promotion as it does on research and development for new treatments.[34]

Given the drug industry's history of aggressive marketing tactics and exorbitant profits, it is clear that this industry is driven by profit and not research and development or saving lives. Big pharma is resistant to change because integrative health will be less lucrative for these companies.

WHERE INTEGRITY BECOMES FUZZY

Reviewing new drug applications is costly, and as a result the U.S. Food and Drug Administration (FDA) was having a difficult time evaluating new drugs in a timely manner. This delay cut into the profits of the pharmaceutical companies, which resulted in the pharmaceutical companies developing a plan that would speed up the process. In 1992 new legislation was passed which allowed the U.S. Government to rely heavily on drug companies to pay the salaries of FDA scientists who reviewed new drug applications.[35] Originally, the sole purpose of this new funding was to speed up the process of having new drugs available. Dr. Jerry Avorn, Professor of Medicine at Harvard Medical School, explained that the legislation required that no part of the funding could be allocated to evaluate side effects of these new drugs after drug approval, which was a time where important safety concerns could arise.[36] Some FDA employees have acknowledged that there is a growing sense that the FDA is accountable to the industry it regulates.[37]

Integrity also becomes fuzzy when individuals who have interests in pharmaceutical companies take positions in government agencies. To avoid this conflict of interest there must be a clear separation between the drug companies and the government agencies that regulate them.[38]

WAITING FOR A CURE?

If you are waiting for a cure, please don't hold your breath. The very system that brings new treatments and drugs to the public has a dif-

ferent motive. Ask yourself: if you were a drug
company, would you make more money curing
someone or treating them for the rest of their
life? Here lies the huge conflict of interest. It
is not in Big Pharma's financial best interest to

> At this time, there is no financial incentive to cure people.

cure us. We expect drug companies to value saving lives over profits,
but this altruism is counter-intuitive to their corporate goals.

Recently, several treatments for cancer have shown great promise
in the pre-clinical phase but because drug companies couldn't patent
the drug, the potential cure was shelved.[39]

One such promising drug is dichloroacetate (DCA). Dr. Evangelos
Michelakis, professor at the University of Alberta Department of Medicine, has shown that DCA causes regression in lung, breast and brain
tumors.[40] This drug is not patentable and is inexpensive to administer,
therefore no drug company will conduct the necessary research.

However, despite the lack of support from the pharmaceutical
industry and thanks to support from the public as well as the University of Alberta and Alberta Health Services, Dr. Michelakis' group has
started human clinical trials.

Intravenous vitamin C therapy may also be a promising cancer
treatment, yet once again this treatment is not patentable and therefore not supported by the pharmaceutical industry. Case reports have
demonstrated regression of tumors without the side effects of chemo
drugs.[41,42] The effectiveness of this therapy is being further studied at
the U.S. National Institute of Health.

How many other promising treatments have been shelved over the
years because profits were not big enough for pharmaceutical companies?

WHO IS RESPONSIBLE?

With active resistance from the pharmaceutical industry, the medical community and the patients themselves, it is challenging to make
necessary changes. Governments are more popular if they give these
groups what they want and don't upset the status quo. All three groups

have played a significant role in the crisis we face today.

Change must take place, and will take place. I believe it is just a matter of time. Will we embrace change that will improve our quality of life and sustain our health care system or we will hit a brick wall?

THE LOSERS

Pharmaceutical companies have been the biggest winners in health care, but who are the biggest losers? We are! Disease trends are on the rise and more of us suffer with chronic illness than ever before. The World Health Organization predicts that deaths caused by diabetes will double between 2005 and 2030.[43] Currently, one in three people have cardiovascular disease, which accounts for 30% of all deaths.[44] Cancer is now a leading cause of death worldwide and the total number of cases globally is increasing. Currently, 1 in every 2.3 men and 1 in every 2.5 women will develop cancer in their lifetime.[45] Autism now affects 1 in 91 children.[46]

4 The Autoimmune Epidemic

We often hear about the three deadly killers: heart disease, cancer and diabetes, but statistically our odds of coming down with an autoimmune disease are much greater! Autoimmune disease occurs when the immune system attacks and damages various parts the body. The following are examples of relatively common autoimmune diseases:

- Celiac
- Inflammatory bowel disease (colitis, Crohn's disease)
- Rheumatoid arthritis
- Psoriasis

- Multiple sclerosis
- Type 1 diabetes
- Asthma

There are over eighty different autoimmune diseases[47] and autoimmune now affects more than 23.5 million people in the U.S. alone.[48] Experts believe that the true number of people who suffer with autoimmune disease could be greater because receiving an accurate diagnosis can be difficult. Autoimmune diseases often share similar symptoms, or their symptoms are common with other health issues.[49] Getting a proper diagnosis can be frustrating and stressful to say the least, as sufferers often move from one expert to the next in hopes of finding an answer to their misery. If you suspect that you have an autoimmune disease, you may have to get a second, third, or even fourth opinion before you receive an accurate diagnosis.[50]

Autoimmune disease can turn lives upside down, either immediately or over time. Autoimmune sufferers often experience a devastating decline in their quality of life, often with debilitating pain, disability and a shortened life.

These diseases also come with a high financial burden. Autoimmune diseases can affect a person's ability to work and are the third leading cause of Social Security disability in the U.S.[51] They require expensive maintenance drugs for the balance of the patient's life.

THE COLD HARD FACTS ON AUTOIMMUNE DISEASES

Over the past 40 years:[52]
- Lupus has almost tripled
- Type 1 diabetes has increased by five times
- Multiple sclerosis (MS) has doubled and even tripled in many countries
- Scleroderma, Crohn's disease, arthritis, autoimmune Addison's disease, and polymyositis have all demonstrated the same alarming increase.

With this dramatic increase in autoimmune disease, doctors are faced with growing patient loads and patients are faced with longer wait times. Why such an epidemic in autoimmune diseases? Experts agree that we are better able to diagnose autoimmune, but this fact alone cannot explain the shocking increase that we are observing. Something in our environment must have changed in the past 50 years... something significant.

> ## So what has changed that's affected our health so greatly?

Although many experts just shrug their shoulders and admit there is no proven explanation for the increased trend in chronic disease, research from around the world is uncovering some big clues. The *increased presence of environmental pollutants* and *the overuse of antibiotics* are two hot topics of study. I have devoted a chapter in this book to environmental toxins, so this topic will be discussed later. I believe that the overuse of antibiotics is largely responsible for the incredible destruction of our health over the past 50 years.

ANTIBIOTICS & DYSBIOSIS

Antibiotics were first introduced in the 1940s and initially were praised as the biggest discovery of the century because of their ability to kill bacterial infections and save lives. In North America, the vast majority of us have taken antibiotics at one time or another; some of us have had the misfortune of taking them repeatedly.

Although antibiotics save many lives, I believe that their overuse is largely responsible for the epidemic of chronic disease that we face today.

It is widely accepted that taking a broad spectrum antibiotic kills the normal flora (good bacteria) in the digestive tract. It is also well understood that side effects of antibiotic include upset stomach, diarrhea and vaginal yeast infections in women.[53] More serious side effects include impaired function of the kidneys, bone marrow, and other organs.

As a consequence of taking antibiotics, we suffer with varying degrees of dysbiosis (disharmony in the digestive tract, or too many bad microbes and not enough good microbes present in the GI tract).

New research is supporting the belief that dysbiosis is a major contributor to the onset of autoimmune disease and chronic disease in general. A recent study by Dr. David J. Margolis et al, researchers at the University of Pennsylvania School of Medicine,[54] considered whether the use of antibiotics (specifically the tetracycline family of antibiotics) for the treatment of acne, could contribute to the development of inflammatory bowel disease (IBD), which includes ulcerative colitis, Crohn's and other diseases of the GI tract. Over 94,000 individuals with a history of acne were interviewed. In this study, 73% of the individuals suffering with IBD, 77% of those suffering with Crohn's disease, and 69% who suffered with colitis had all been treated for acne in the past with the tetracycline class of antibiotics.

An earlier study by the same researchers found that we are two times more likely to contract an upper respiratory tract infection within the first year of taking antibiotics for acne than if we chose not to take the antibiotics.[55]

Table 2. Association between the use of tetracycline class antimicrobial for at least one month and the incidence of individuals with inflammatory bowel disease (IBD), Crohn's disease or ulcerative colitis

Disease	Overall number of individuals in the study with the disease	Number of individuals that used antibiotics for acne	Number of individuals that did not use antibiotics for acne	Likelihood of developing the disease after antibiotic use for acne (%)	Likelihood of developing the disease: antibiotics not used for acne (%)
IBD	207	152	55	73%	27%
Crohn's disease	71	55	16	77%	23%
Ulcerative colitis	99	68	31	69%	31%

*Modified from: Margolis, Fanelli, Hoffstad, and Lewis. (2010).

Researchers at the University of Nottingham found an association between the onset of Crohn's disease and the use of antibiotics 2–5 years before diagnosis.[56] This research further supports the notion that the use of antibiotics can increase one's risk of inflammatory bowel disease.

The growing epidemic of digestive disease in North America is a major concern. In the U.S. alone, 95 million Americans experience digestive problems, and more than 10 million of these people are hospitalized each year, at a total cost of more than $40 billion annually.[57] The Canadian Digestive Health Foundation reported that:[58]

- At least 60% or 20 million Canadians suffer with a digestive disease which accounts for about $18 billion in health care costs and lost productivity.
- Canada has one of highest incidence rates for digestive disease in the world, and in particular irritable bowel syndrome.
- Canada has the highest incidence of gastrointestinal ulcers in the world.

Researchers from the University of Washington found that increasing the number of days on antibiotics and increasing the number of antibiotic prescriptions were associated with an increased risk of breast cancer and increased mortality rates due to breast cancer. This was true for all classes of antibiotics.[59]

It will take many peer reviewed studies to convince the medical community that antibiotics have a dark side. The government can't afford to fund this research; pharmaceutical companies won't fund this research. Therefore, if you want to wait for this to be scientifically proven you will probably have to wait a very long time.

ANTIBIOTICS: TOO MUCH KILLING GOING ON

There is a saying that "disease or death begins in the gut." I believe that this statement holds much truth.

We take antibiotics to kill the infections which make us sick.

Unfortunately, the antibiotics we take not only kill our infections, but also kill off the good bacteria that live inside our digestive tract.[60] The presence of good bacteria is the body's natural defense to control and contain the growth of unwanted parasites and pathogens. Once this delicate balance has been disturbed we forfeit the natural defense that protects us and we are now vulnerable to the overgrowth of parasites and pathogens—in particular fungi.

In summary, if we know that taking antibiotics destroys our natural defenses which leads to an overgrowth of fungi and other bad microbes (which the side effects of antibiotics confirms), do we really have to wait for the experts to prove that the overuse of antibiotics is a major contributor to the prevalence of digestive disease today? It's your choice—to wait for the experts to spell this out for you many years from now, or you can choose to take charge of your health and try a safe approach. What do you have to lose?

If your doctor recommends that you should take an antibiotic, you should follow the advice. But if you want to avoid using them in the future, then *it is your responsibility to restore the natural defenses in your GI tract and improve the strength of your immune system* so that you will rarely (if ever) need to use antibiotics again in the future. This book will show you how to accomplish this.

5 The Perfect Storm of Healthcare

So what if we just bury our heads in the sand and carry on with the status quo, knowing full well that cold hard facts are telling us that disease trends and health care costs are rising at an unsustainable rate. If we continue down this path, what's ahead?

In Canada, we are already experiencing higher taxes and longer wait times, but this is just the beginning: the money that is required to sustain this system will have to come from somewhere.

Nicholas Webb makes the following predictions in his book *The Cost of Being Sick:*[61]

1. *Disease trends will continue to rise affecting younger age groups.*

The Canadian Heart and Stroke foundation's 2010 annual report[62] warns of an impending crisis. Between 1994 and 2005 high blood pressure rates among Canadians skyrocketed 77%, diabetes by 45% and obesity by 18%. In the age group of 35 to 49 years of age, high blood pressure increased 127%, diabetes 64% and obesity by 29%. Even more disturbing is the 261% increase in high blood pressure in our Canadian teens—as young as 12 years old—and young adults during this same period of time. Young adults have now been officially designated as one of Canada's newest at-risk groups for heart disease. The Heart and Stroke Foundation warns that "these increases will translate into an explosion of heart disease in the next generation."[63]

2. *Employees will feel the squeeze on their paychecks as they pay for increased health care premiums that employers refuse to cover.*

In the U.S. in 2010, health care premiums rose by 10% and this entire increase was passed on to employees. Over the past five years, health care premium costs in the U.S. rose by 47% while the average wage increase was 18%.[64]

3. *Health care costs will become the new mortgage.*

Could you imagine paying $1000/month for health care for a single person or $2000/month for a family? That would equate to $12,000–$24,000/year for health care. These numbers may seem unrealistic, yet in the U.S. in 2009, approximately 23% of adults were already paying these rates for individual or family health care coverage. As health care premiums continue to increase more people will forgo needed care and will opt out of carrying health care insurance[65] which will reduce the effectiveness of the health care system.

4. Health score dictates premiums.

Life insurance companies rate our health to determine if we qualify for life insurance and decide what our premiums will be. Webb predicts that Americans will soon be rated by health care insurance companies on the level of their health. Health insurance companies will consider medical history, genetics, age, gender, race, body fat, occupation, and other personal health related factors.[66] If your health score is low, you may pay a higher premium or you may be denied health insurance.

Several companies are implementing this already. Some employers offer cash bonuses to employees who fill out health risk assessments, who do not smoke, or who participate in wellness programs.[67]

I know what Canadian readers are thinking to themselves at this moment: "In Canada we have universal health care and therefore we are not victim to the tactics of the health insurance companies in the U.S." The fact is, we too must pay these rising health care costs one way or another, whether through increased taxes and wait times, user fees, or some combination of both.

I am not a pessimist and my goal isn't to depress you with all these stats. I do, however, want to make it blatantly clear that our approach to health care is not working. There is a better way—and for the balance of the book I will focus on the solution.

The biggest challenges we face are shifting our beliefs around health care and reallocating billions of health care dollars to support a more balanced, preventative and integrative approach to maintaining the system we have in place. And as we have seen, there is fiery opposition to this approach.

You, however, don't have to wait for these imminent changes to the system. My hope is that *you* will choose to become a Wellness Champion, embrace the necessary changes and decrease your dependence on our unsustainable health care system. This book is written to empower you to take responsibility for your health and improve your quality of life. You don't have to wait, you can begin today!

THE CONFUSION

When I have coached clients in wellness over the years, I have observed an all-too-common frustration and genuine confusion as people desperately seek ways to improve their quality of life. There are literally thousands of natural products on the market, all claiming to be the answer to our woes. Many people try supplements and therapies one after another, in a desperate hope to find an answer. Each time we don't find the answer, we become a little less hopeful that we will ever find a solution. It is disheartening to see people spend hundreds or thousands of dollars on therapies and supplements only to experience limited results, if any. Governments are not able to protect us from fraudulent claims made by these companies.

My goal is to provide you with a basic understanding of what is required for optimal health so that you are better able to decide if something will benefit you or if it is just marketing hype. Yes, it is important to eat right, exercise, drink lots of water and get your beauty sleep, but there is another very significant piece of the wellness puzzle that has been missing. I believe that this virtually unknown component of wellness (see page 85) plays a major role in why our health is breaking down at such an alarming rate. Although interest is growing and many research papers have been published on this topic, it is not currently recognized by the majority of the medical and scientific communities. This book includes many references reviewed by scientific peers so that the skeptics can research this topic further.

THE BLUEPRINT OF WELLNESS

The blueprint of your wellness plan is made up of four pillars. Once you understand the Four Pillars of Wellness, you will be pleasantly surprised that the concept is quite simple. You will see that it makes perfect sense. I encourage you to use common sense and your intuition when searching for solutions. If an expert tells you something and it doesn't sit right with you, ask for clarification. If you are still not peaceful about it, get another opinion. Experts are human and no one knows your body better than you. You must take responsibility for your health!

The Four Pillars of Wellness

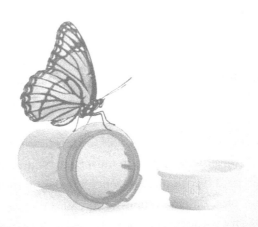

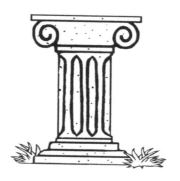

Pillar #1
Optimize Nutrition

NUTRITION IS THE FOUNDATION FOR WELLNESS

Optimizing nutrition is the first pillar of wellness because it lays a strong foundation for wellness. The body is a miracle. It is made up of at least one hundred trillion cells and each cell performs millions of chemical reactions. Healthy cells build healthy tissues, glands and organs. Nutrients from our food are vital for cells to grow, multiply, renew and perform necessary chemical reactions every day. The body has the innate ability to heal itself and optimal nutrition provides the fuel to support this. Therefore, optimizing nutrition must be the foundation for wellness.

> Optimizing nutrition is the foundation for wellness.

Nutritional deficiencies will limit the success of therapies, hinder wellness and cause disease. A person might try complementary therapies such as chelation, acupuncture, chiropractic therapy, massage, etc., but will likely experience only limited benefits if underlying nutritional deficiencies are not recognized and corrected. If the body is supported with optimal nutrition it can and will do much of the repairing and healing on its own, and any additional therapies will be more effective. Table 3 demonstrates several examples of diseases caused by specific vitamin deficiencies.

Table 3. Vitamin and mineral deficiencies and their associated diseases

Vitamin/Mineral	Deficiency/Disease
Vitamin A	Night blindness
Vitamin C	Scurvy
Vitamin B12	Pernicious anemia
Vitamin D	Rickets, osteoporosis
Vitamin B3/Niacin	Pellagra
Calcium	Rickets in children, osteomalacia and osteoporosis in adults
Iron	Anemia
Omega 3 fats	Cardiovascular disease

Although we live in the land of plenty, our dependence on processed foods, together with the decline of nutrients in our food, puts us at risk of nutritional deficiencies now more than ever before.

As we optimize nutrition by returning to whole foods and include food-form supplements that fill in the gaps of what is missing from our diet, we will experience:

- More energy
- A stronger immune system
- A greater sense of well-being
- Improved mood
- Improved ability to handle stress
- Improved sleep
- Improved brain function
- Success in finally reaching our ideal body shape and maintaining it

The Problem

WHAT HAPPENED TO OUR FOOD?

Have you ever picked a vine-ripened tomato from a garden? Do you remember that amazing smell—and that taste! The smell and the flavours of vine-ripened produce boast of their phytonutrient content. Now think of that blotchy, whitish-red colored tomato from the produce department of your grocery store in the dead of winter. The field tomato is firm and it doesn't have that amazing smell. As you cut it open you notice the whitish fibrous texture inside, and as you eat it you notice a distinct lack of flavour. You just paid close to $4/lb for something that tastes like nothing.

On your next trip to the grocery store, you chose the softer, redder hothouse tomato. Unlike the field tomato, it does possess the faint smell of a real tomato, but later on at home when you eat it, you realize the flavor is not much better than the field variety; the hothouse variety was a bit cheaper than the field tomatoes so at least you saved a buck or two.

Green bananas and hard avocados turn brown inside before they ever ripen. You find celery that has been in your crisper for weeks and still looks the same as the day you bought it: how is that possible? You have to buy baby carrots because the big carrots are bitter and sometimes taste just plain nasty. Rock hard kiwis can sit on the kitchen counter for two weeks and still be hard enough to use as a puck in a good game of street hockey. It just isn't fun eating veggies anymore.

You know that you are supposed to eat at least five to nine servings of vegetables and fruit each day, but it is quite a chore to eat them let alone pay for them. They lack wholesome flavour and color. It seems that you aren't getting the value for the price you pay... it seems that much of the produce is itself sick.

So what has happened to our produce?

According to the experts, the nutrient content in our produce has dropped dramatically over the past 50 years. Here's why.

MALNOURISHED IN THE LAND OF PLENTY

Genetic modification, intensive same-crop farming, green harvest practices (harvesting produce before it ripens), and long storage times have all played a part in reducing the nutrient content in our produce, which has resulted in fruits and vegetables that lack flavor and appeal.

IT ALL STARTS WITH NOT-SO-HEALTHY SOIL

Soil is the starting point of the human food chain: soil fertility impacts human health. Plants require many minerals from the soil. In plant production, trace mineral deficiencies are a common nutritional concern when talking about food crops.[68] The health of a crop will be negatively impacted if certain minerals in the soil are either deficient or present at toxic levels. Soils become depleted of trace minerals if the same crops are planted throughout the year, year after year. Synthetic commercial fertilizers do not contain all the trace minerals naturally found in the soil and therefore cannot properly replenish it. So if the same crops are grown continuously, certain trace minerals are at risk of becoming depleted.

Just as some minerals can become depleted with continuous same-crop farming, other trace minerals can build up and cause toxicity in growing plants, which can then be transferred to consumers and also degrade the quality of water downstream.[69]

The overuse of synthetic NPK (nitrogen phosphorus potassium) fertilizers can affect the fertility of the soil by damaging microbes that free up essential minerals.[70] Trace minerals have also become depleted with the increased use of NPK synthetic commercial fertilizers that do not contain trace minerals.[71]

The fertility and health of our soil is also compromised as hazardous industrial wastes are recycled into fertilizers. Several dozen toxic metals like lead and mercury have been introduced into our farmland, lawns, and garden soils for years. In the U.S., between 1990 and 1996, six hundred companies from 44 different states sent 270 million pounds of toxic waste to farms and fertilizer companies across the country.[72] One study tested twenty-nine fertilizers and found that they all contained twenty-two toxic heavy metals. These toxic heavy metals contaminate our soils and are linked to ecological and human health hazards.[73]

Chang and Page reported that "the harmful effects caused by trace elements tend to be chronic, gradually building up over continual exposures. As a result, potential ecological and human-health consequences related to the release of trace elements may go on unnoticed."[74]

So why are governments allowing companies to dispose toxic waste in this manner? Good question. This is a great reason to go organic.

> **"Farmers get paid by the weight of a crop, not by amount of nutrients," says Dr. Ronald Davis, biochemist at the University of Texas at Austin.**

IS BIGGER REALLY BETTER?

Farming is a competitive industry and therefore farmers benefit from selecting plants that grow faster and produce bigger yields. As a result, most farmers choose varieties that do just that. Unfortunately, faster-grown produce doesn't have as much time to develop the same nutrient concentrations as traditional plants, and this is detrimental for the consumer.[75]

Bigger yields equal greater profit. But as crop yields increase, the ability of the plant to extract, utilize and transport minerals from the soil, and its ability to synthesize proteins, vitamins and other nutrients, all decrease.

WHAT IS GREEN HARVEST?

Most of us depend on produce from California, Mexico, South America or some other distant country for a good part of the year. This produce is picked green and not allowed to ripen on the vine. Green bananas and rock hard avocados and kiwis are examples of this. Green produce has a longer shelf life so it won't rot while being shipped from the farm to the store; and it will last longer on the store shelf. This equates to less waste and more profit for the wholesalers and retailers.

> As crop yields increase, the concentrations of minerals and protein decrease— a genetic dilution effect.

This all sounds great in theory, but is this good for us? Research shows that there is a big downside to green harvest. Most fruits and vegetables reach their full phytonutrient and vitamin content when they are ripe. Picking produce before it is ripe can significantly compromise its vitamin content.[77] Dr. Anne-Berit Wold et al[78] found that "the ripening stage influences the total antioxidant capacity in tomatoes... green unripe tomatoes contain consistently less antioxidants than the ripe fruits."

PEPPERS FROM WHERE?

Another reason for the drop in nutrients in our produce is due to the fact that our fruits and veggies have usually been in transport for at least a week before we purchase them. In our local grocery store we can buy beans, tomatoes, and mangos from Mexico, pineapples from Costa Rica, kiwis from New Zealand, and peppers from Spain. The produce department has become an international marketplace. This gives us a tremendous amount of variety, but the quality with respect to nutrient content is often questionable.

"There is a rapid drop in nutrients when produce has been stored for more than a few days. When it hits the refrigerator it can lose up to 50% of its vitamin C and other nutrient content in the following week, depending on the temperature," says Dr. Barbara P. Klein, Professor of Food Science and Human Nutrition at the University of Illinois, Urbana-Champaign.[79]

JUST HOW SERIOUS IS THE DECLINE IN NUTRIENTS?

- In 1951, a woman would have to eat two peaches a day to receive the U.S. recommended daily allowance of vitamin A. Today that number has increased to *fifty three peaches.*[80]
- Nine oranges today will provide the same amount of vitamin A that your grandparents got from just one orange.[81]

Dr. Anne-Marie Mayer[82] compared 20 fruits and 20 vegetables grown in the 1930s and the 1980s and found several marked reductions in mineral content. Three other studies found a 5%–40% or more decline in certain minerals in produce, and a fourth study showed a significant decrease in vitamins and protein.[83]

Because of the dramatic decline in nutrient content in our produce, the USDA[84] increased their recommendations for daily servings of fruits and vegetables to 9–13 servings per day (depending on energy expenditure). Yet less than 18% of the population is even following the daily recommended servings of 5–9 fruits and vegetables from the Food Pyramid.[85]

Although the sad state of our food may seem disheartening, it is important to remember that vegetables and fruits are still our most nutrient dense food and we must consume them for optimal health. As we become more aware and educated about what is happening to our food and why, we can make better choices. The consumer drives the market. As we demand produce that is rich in nutrients and free of toxic chemicals, a greater selection of more nutritious produce will be available for us.

THE BODY IS NOT STUPID!

I will always remember the honesty of my cell biology professor who confessed that what he was about to teach us was science's best understanding of how the cell functioned. He admitted that some of the information that he would teach us might be disproven in the future.

Science may have a limited understanding of how the human body works, but it has been my experience that the body is perfectly capable of healing and repairing itself if given the correct nutrients and support. *If this is true, then doesn't it make sense to try to support the body naturally so it can do what it was designed to do before we resort to toxic drugs? What a simple concept!*

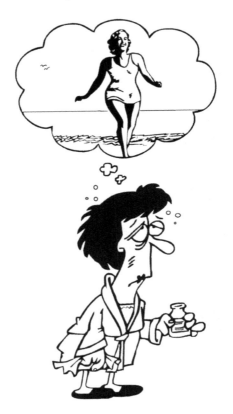

When did we stop using common sense?
Was it after years of influence from drug companies
who enlightened us that we need their drugs
to suppress our immune systems?

Nutrition & Supplements in a Nutshell

1. REGULARLY EAT WHOLE-FOOD MEALS

What type of food does the body really need?

Our body needs real food. Whole food must be our main source of nutrients as it provides a variety of nutrients, enzymes (if raw), water, and fiber. Whole foods are in their natural state. We have become so accustomed to eating processed foods that many of us have forgotten what real food is (see Table 4).

Table 4. Real food vs. processed food

Examples of Whole Foods (close to natural state)	Examples of Processed Foods
Sprouted wheat bread	White bread, brown bread
Wild rice, brown rice: long grain, short grain, basmati	White rice, instant rice, converted white and brown rice, parboiled rice
Fresh fruit	Fruit cups, fruit juice, fruit rollups
Grass fed organic beef, wild fish, organic chicken	Luncheon sandwich meats, pepperoni, sausage, fast food burgers
Whole raw nuts	Hydrogenated peanut butter
Natural honey, maple syrup	High fructose corn syrup
Baked potato	French fries

Eat 9–13 servings of produce each day

The USDA now recommends 9–13 servings of fruits and veggies each day, depending on how much energy we burn. Make a conscious effort to eat as many different fruits and veggies as you can and be sure to vary the types and colors of produce you eat. Buy local when available and certified organic if possible. It is vital to keep track of how many servings you are getting. Plan your meals ahead and keep your fridge stocked with veggies. People under high levels of stress (physical, mental or emotional) will require more nutrients.

> **All that man needs for health and healing has been provided by God in nature; the challenge of science is to find it.**
> Paracelsus (1493–1541)

Go for variety
Eat a variety of whole foods each day. Create a rainbow of colors on your plate. Remember that variety offers an array of nutrients. If you eat the same foods day after day you will run the risk of becoming deficient in certain nutrients.

Buy certified organic and local food when possible
Certified organic and local foods are usually more nutritious. In addition, certified organic foods are grown without synthetic pesticides and fertilizers, do not contain genetically modified organisms and are not processed using irradiation, industrial solvents or chemical additives.[86] Be aware that organic and certified organic are not the same thing. The certified organic industry is heavily regulated. A farmer can call their product natural or organic and this may be true, but only *certified organic* producers are regulated. When buying organic food from a producer you are relying on the trust factor.

As you shop for whole food, use common sense. If it is the dead of winter and a certain vegetable is labeled certified organic but it looks pathetically sick, it is probably not worth purchasing even though it is certified organic. Select food that looks healthy.

Local farmers have the luxury of allowing produce to ripen longer on the vine. Local produce is often picked the day it is sold and thus has much more flavor and contains a significantly higher nutrient content than produce that is picked green and has been in transport for a week or more before we purchase it. Grow a garden, visit local farms, and patronize farmers' markets as often as possible.

Because small doses of pesticide chemicals and other environmental chemicals can cause long term damage to our health,[87] it should be our goal to minimize the amount of environmental chemicals that we ingest from our food and water. Certified organic food can help reduce our exposure to pesticide chemicals.

Most people cannot afford to buy all of their food certified organic. Also, certified organic food is not always readily available. A great way to start making better choices is to use the *Environmental Working Group's Shopper's Guide to Pesticides* (Table 5). Eating non-certified

Table 5. *Environmental Working Group's 2011 Shopper's Guide to Pesticides*[89]

The Dirty Dozen (Highest Pesticide Load)	The Clean Fifteen (Lowest Pesticide Load)
Celery	Onions
Peaches	Avocado
Strawberries	Sweet Corn
Apples	Pineapples
Blueberries	Mangoes
Nectarines (Imported)	Sweet Peas
Sweet Bell Peppers	Asparagus
Spinach	Kiwi
Lettuce	Cabbage
Kale/Collard Greens	Eggplant
Potatoes	Cantaloupe
Grapes (Imported)	Watermelon
	Grapefruits
	Mushrooms
	Sweet Potato

*Modified from the *Environmental Working Group's Shopper's Guide to Pesticides* www.ewg.org

organic produce from the Clean Fifteen group and avoiding produce that is not certified organic from the Dirty Dozen group will significantly lower a person's ingested pesticide load.[88]

2. USE REAL-FOOD DIETARY SUPPLEMENTS TO FILL IN WHAT IS MISSING IN YOUR FOOD

Although plant-sourced nutritional supplements are important to fill in what's missing from our food, they cannot provide all the nutrients found in whole food. Thus we should never use supplements as a substitute, but instead use them to enrich our whole-food eating plan.

You will experience the greatest benefits to your health if you include standardized, natural plant-based vitamins, minerals, antioxidants, phytosterols, phytonutrients, glyconutrients, and essential fatty acids in your dietary supplements. So what are these things?

Science has discovered that our bodies need at least nine different groups of nutrients for optimal health. These include carbohydrates, amino acids, essential fatty acids (good fats), vitamins, minerals, antioxidants, glyconutrients, phytosterols (plant hormones), and many phytonutrients. Most of us are aware of the importance of vitamins, minerals, antioxidants and essential fats, and realize that we aren't getting enough from our food. Phytochemicals, phytosterols and glyconutrients are also important nutrients that many people are not as familiar with.

Phytochemicals

Phytonutrients or phytochemicals are plant nutrients that benefit human health. Over twelve thousand phytochemicals have been discovered, but only a few have been studied. Table 6 shows examples of various produce and some of their phytochemical content. These nutrients play an important role in how the body uses vitamins and minerals, neutralizing free radicals and protecting us from diabetes, cancer, heart disease, stroke and many other serious conditions. It is important to choose a rainbow of colours when you eat vegetables and fruits because produce of various colours each offer different phytochemicals.

Table 6. Phytochemicals in food

Phytochemical	Food Source	Color(s)	Possible Benefits
Carotenoids: Alpha-Carotene, Beta-Carotene, Beta-Cryptoxanthin, Lycopene, Lutein, and Zeaxanthin	Carrots, Tomatoes, Pumpkin, Spinach, Kale, Okra, Cantaloupe, Watermelon	Yellow, Orange, and Red Pigments	Neutralize free radicals, reduce risk of cardiovascular disease, and some cancers
Anthocyanins: Cyanidin, Delphinidin, Malvidin, Pelargonidin, Peonidin, Petunidin	Berries: Strawberries, Blueberries, Raspberries, etc.	Red, Blue, Purple	Improve vision, decreased blood clotting, reduce risk of chronic disease
Sulfides, Thiols	Garlic, Onions, Leeks, Olives, Scallions	White, Green, Black	Decrease LDL cholesterol, protect against gastric and colorectal cancer
Sulforaphane	Broccoli, Kale, Cabbage, Cauliflower and other cruciferous vegetables	Green, White	Neutralize free radicals, reduce risk of some cancers

Modified from: Linus Pauling Institute, 2010, Heneman, Zidenberg, 2007

Phytosterols

Our endocrine system produces over 87 different hormones and is responsible for energy levels, mood, sexual function, metabolic rate, fat metabolism, quality of sleep, immune function, body temperature and blood sugar regulation. Phytosterols are plant substances that are very similar to hormones or hormone precursors. Our bodies use phytosterols along with other nutrients to produce a healthy balance of hormones. The body is genetically programmed to produce the right amount of each type of hormone.

Earlier human diets (which were more plant based) were rich in phytosterols whereas the typical North American diet is deficient. Today most people are not getting adequate amounts of these nutrients from the food they eat. Studies have demonstrated that diets rich in phytosterols are associated with decreased risk of cancer, decreased serum LDL cholesterol and improved urinary tract function.[90] The highest concentrations of these nutrients are found in unrefined vegetables, nut and olive oils. Nuts, seeds, whole grains, legumes, beets, Brussels sprouts, cabbage, yams, oranges, apples and bananas are also great sources of phytosterols. Doesn't it make good sense to provide your body with adequate amounts of these nutrients so that your body can build the proper balance of hormones that it is designed to produce? Why not try incorporating more of these foods into your life? Phytosterols do not have the undesirable side effect of synthetic hormones and steroids

> "Currently, over twelve thousand phytochemicals have been discovered..."

Glyconutrients—the Best Kept Secret in Nutrition

The Greek word *Glyco* means sugar or sweet. Glyconutrients are simple sugars, not to be confused with sucrose or table sugar. In the human body these simple sugars are attached to lipids (fats) and proteins and have very special jobs. They were first described in 1734, and then again in 1865.[91] Although this field of study has had a slow start, interest began to grow in the 1960s and then really took off in the 1980s. Because most of the research has been done in the last 20+ years, most people are not familiar with this important and unique class of nutrients. In the year 2000, I graduated with a science degree in biology and was never introduced to them. I was taught that antibodies, hormones, and enzymes were all proteins when in fact they are glycoproteins. They all have a very important sugar component to them.

The Eight Glyconutrients

These simple sugars are called monosaccharides: mono meaning *one* and saccharide meaning *sugar*. A monosaccharide is the smallest unit of a carbohydrate, just as an amino acid is the smallest unit of a protein. Science has discovered about 200 monosaccharides in nature, of which eight are commonly involved in how our cells communicate with each other.[92] These eight glyconutrients essentially make up the alphabet for the language of our cells. Not only are they a very important functional part of antibodies, collagen, various hormones, enzymes, and other constituents in the body, they are also found on the surface of the cell.[93] On the surface of the cell they are attached to each other in a specific order and resemble bead-like chains or branches. Communication between cells takes place at these branches. If even one of these simple sugars is missing on a branch, miscommunication can occur.

To better understand the importance of glyconutrients, consider the human blood types. The difference between type A, B and O blood is the presence or absence of just one simple sugar at the end of a short chain attached to the red blood cell. If someone with type A blood is given type B blood, the immune cells would recognize this very slight difference and the result could be fatal.

Glyconutrients support optimal immune function, brain function, hormonal regulation, metabolism, digestive health, fertilization, and many other functions in the body.

So where are these nutrients found? It starts with mother's breast milk which contains 5 of the 8 simple sugars. Table 7 shows various sources of glyconutrients. This list is not all-inclusive but it does show that in order to maintain wellness, eating a variety of foods is very important. As with other nutrients, most people are not getting enough glyconutrients from their food.

Table 7. Sources of glyconutrients

Glyconutrient	Sources
Mannose	Aloe vera (acemannan is a chain of mannose molecules), kelp, shiitake mushroom, ground fenugreek, guar gum, black currants, red currants, gooseberries, green beans, cabbage, tomatoes, turnip
Galactose	Dairy products, legumes (dried beans and peas), small amounts in artichoke, mushroom, olive and peanut, papaya, bell pepper, tomato, watermelons
Fucose	Seaweed (kelp and wakane)
N-acetylglucosamine	Shiitake mushroom, shark cartilage, beef cartilage, glucosamine sulphate, algae
Glucose	Many naturally ripened vegetables and fruits, honey
N-acetylgalactosamine	Shark cartilage, beef cartilage, chondroitin sulphate, red algae
N-acetylneuraminic acid	Whey protein concentrate or isolate, chicken eggs
Xylose	Kelp, ground psyllium seeds, guava, pears, blackberries, loganberries, raspberries, Aloe vera, broccoli, spinach, eggplant, peas, green beans, okra, cabbage, corn

The study of these simple sugars in the body has been touted as the biggest discovery in the past hundred years in nutrition. Many universities worldwide now study glycobiology, and thousands of scientific papers have been published on this subject since the early 1980s.

Glycomics, the study of the structure and function of these nutrients in the body, has been identified as "one of the top ten emerging technologies that will change the world" by a leading research institute.[94]

If the discovery of glyconutrients is so great, why are we not hearing about this in the media? I have been supplementing with these nutrients for the past 10 years and they are the last supplement that I would give up. They have made a big impact on my quality of life. It saddens me that most people don't know that they exist and even if they have heard about them they don't really understand their significance.

Pharmaceutical companies are attempting to recreate these nutrients in the lab. Their hope is to make synthetic versions and attach them to their drugs to make new, more effective maintenance products. It is much more cost effective for companies to produce synthetic versions vs. extracting them from plants, but this is not necessarily better for us because synthetic chemical versions of nutrients are not recognized and used by the body as effectively as nutrients from plants. Also, it is more lucrative to make a synthetic version because natural plant nutrients cannot be patented. Add to this the fact that manufacturing these special sugars in the lab is very challenging due to their complex structure, and considering all these factors, the general public is simply not learning about this very important class of nutrients at this time.

The discovery of glyconutrients has also been the most controversial and disruptive issue in nutritional science in the past 100 years. The debate revolves around the following: some scientists believe that the body is able to make all eight simple sugars and that there is no proof that it needs to receive them from our diet. They also believe that there is no benefit to supplementing the diet with these nutrients. In the other camp are thousands of ecstatic people, including myself, who have experienced a significant improvement in our health after taking these nutrients. It didn't matter to us what the scientists were claiming. Because this food nutrient is completely safe and we have personally experienced significant benefits in the quality of our lives, we are prepared to continue taking the supplement.

In recent years several scientific studies have shown very impressive findings, discrediting the negative opponents in the debate. Supplementing with a specific glyconutrient blend demonstrated a significant improvement in memory and cognitive function,[95] improved visual discrimination and working memory,[96] enhanced brainwave frequencies known to be associated with attention or alertness[97], and improved mental reaction time and enhanced concentration.[98]

Further research presented at the 2009 Jenner Glycobiology Symposium in Brussels, Belgium, showed that supplementing with the same glyconutrient mixture affects specific genes that help modulate the immune system and that the glyconutrients are in fact absorbed and used by the body.[99] This new research is embraced by many scientists because it is based on changes in the structure and function of the cell and not mere anecdotal case reports.

Although these initial findings are impressive and consistent with the experiences of many grateful people, more research is needed to help us better understand how and why these nutrients benefit human health. I agree with recently retired award-winning U.S. Trademark and Patent official, Dr. John Rollins, who stated that "...integrative health may be an industry-saving strategy for health care, and glyconutrients may be the best technology to support that change."[100] I am hopeful that more research will be done in this field, not necessarily to make more effective pharmaceuticals, but to improve our understanding of the function of glyconutrients in the body and why so many have experienced such wonderful improvements to their quality of life. Are these great benefits the result of correcting a nutritional deficiency? Is it merely a lack of these nutrients in our diet or are other factors involved?

> "Integrative health may be an industry saving strategy for health care, and glyconutrients may be the best technology to support that change."
>
> — Dr. John Rollins.

We have discussed three groups of nutrients that are less understood: phytochemicals, phytosterols and glyconutrients. Yet there are thousands of nutrients that our bodies need for optimal health—some we have yet to discover. At this point you may be feeling slightly overwhelmed, thinking "I thought this stuff was going to be simplified for me." Bear with me—I promise to do just that.

WHY DO I NEED TO TAKE SUPPLEMENTS?

There are three main reasons why the majority of people need to take nutritional supplements. Firstly, most of us do not eat enough fruits and vegetables each day to support optimal health. Secondly, much of the produce we eat is lacking in nutrients, unless you are fortunate enough to live in a climate that allows you to have a garden year round. Finally, many of us need to supplement because we suffer with some degree of dysbiosis (disharmony in the digestive tract).

In general, dysbiosis occurs when the microbes that live in the digestive tract are out of balance. The good or friendly bacteria that should be present in great numbers have been reduced, while the population of bad bugs (parasites) that compete for our nutrients are great in number. If parasites thrive in our body, they rob us of important nutrients. These bad bugs also cause inflammation and damage the lining of the GI tract which hinders our absorption of nutrients from our food. Dysbiosis is very common in North America, mostly due to the overuse of antibiotics, corticosteroids, and oral contraceptives. Dysbiosis will be discussed in depth within this book.

I ALREADY EAT A HEALTHY DIET!

From my years of coaching, I have come to realize that what people believe is a nutritious eating plan is very subjective and varies considerably from one person to the next. Each person has his or her own perspective on what healthy eating is. Also, most people do not take the time to prepare whole-food meals from scratch but instead rely on processed foods for meals and/or snacks. Despite the fact that obesity is epidemic, the government predicts a continued growing demand for convenient processed foods.

As a result, most of us are not getting enough essential nutrients to keep our bodies working at their best. How can we expect the body to carry out thousands of reactions each day if it doesn't have the required fuel? It is truly amazing how accommodating the human body is. Many people live on processed food for years before they are diagnosed with disease. Our bodies will put up with much abuse, but only for so long. How long would your car run if you put a can of Coke in it each day?

SYNERGY: ONE PLUS ONE DOES NOT ALWAYS EQUAL TWO!

It is important to re-emphasize that a person cannot pop any single supplement and get all the nutrition they need to enjoy vibrant health. But a whole-food eating plan together with supplementation is beneficial and necessary for most of us.

We know that the body is designed to get nutrients from food, and that optimal nutrition supports optimal structure and function in the body. Synergy occurs with plant-sourced nutrients because the benefit received from the combination of plant nutrients is greater than the sum of their individual benefits.

> "It is foolish to think you can pop any single supplement and get all the nutrition you need to enjoy vibrant health."

It may be tempting to try one synthetic vitamin at a time in hopes of finding a deficiency, but the truth is that many nutrients work together for a greater benefit. We may have adopted the mentality of a one vitamin cure for one disease from our experience with pharmaceuticals.

Plant-sourced vitamins are not isolated in nature but are found in a complex with other plant nutrients. "It is the combination of these plant nutrients with vitamins that create food synergy," says Dr. Susan Taylor Mayne, a professor at the Yale School of Public Health's Division of Chronic Disease Epidemiology.[101]

Natural vitamin C is not ascorbic acid

Vitamin C in fruit is not just ascorbic acid. It exists as a complex of nutrients which includes bioflavonoids, rutin, ascorbigen, factor J, factor K, factor P, tyrosinase, ascorbic acid and other components. The chemical isolate ascorbic acid only makes up a small percent of the total vitamin C complex found in food.

So why are most supplements made with or from ascorbic acid?

Because it is cheaper to synthesize vitamins in a laboratory from chemicals than to extract them from plants and, until recently, the existing technologies would have produced a very large pill to swallow if produced from plant sources.

> **Synergy—many nutrients work together for a greater combined benefit.**

Expensive urine?

In the past, many doctors believed that taking vitamins resulted in what they called expensive urine. They argued that the body absorbs a very small percentage of synthetic nutrients and the rest is just waste. Although this is true, a survey taken in 2007 showed that more than 70% of all doctors and 80% of all nurses in the U.S. both use and recommend supplements to their patients.[102] Also, an article in the June 2002 issue of the *Journal of the American Medical Association* (JAMA) stated, "Most people do not consume an optimal amount of all vitamins by diet alone ... It appears prudent for all adults to take vitamin supplements."

If adults aren't getting enough nutrients from the food they are eating, then what about our children? Could it be that children are also deficient in nutrients? Isn't optimal nutrition even more important for them as their bodies are actively growing?

Optimizing nutrition in children will improve their memory, mood, and ability to focus and learn, and will strengthen their immune systems. As a teacher, I have seen remarkable improvements in the attention, focus, and alertness of some of my students after their parents decided to optimize their children's nutrition with whole foods and plant-based supplements. Good nutrition offers many benefits and no side effects.

SYNTHETIC VITAMINS

Most vitamins were discovered early in the twentieth century. As science discovered that deficiencies in vitamins and minerals could lead to disease, the recommended daily allowance (RDA) was created. The RDA is the amount of each essential nutrient that our body needs each day to work optimally and thus stay healthy.

The first vitamin supplements were synthetic, which means that they were made from chemicals such as petroleum and coal-tar derivatives in a laboratory and not from food. Synthetic vitamins are isolated chemical substances.

Synthetic vitamins have been the norm for many years because they provide some benefits, are inexpensive to produce compared to plant vitamins, and are easy to standardize.

> **Most vitamin/mineral supplements sold today are synthetic.**

Standardizing supplements is important because the consumer is able to determine the amount of each nutrient that is present in the supplement so they know what they are paying for. The quantities of synthetic vitamins or minerals in the supplement are usually listed as milligrams (mg) or international units (IU).

Disadvantages of synthetic vitamins

Since the body is designed to get its nutrition from real food, synthetic versions of vitamins are not fully absorbed and used by the body as food nutrients. Most of the synthetic vitamin passes through the body and goes down the toilet, hence the term expensive urine. In fact, some research has shown that high doses of certain synthetic vitamins may actually be harmful to our health as they can cause deficiencies in other nutrients and also an increased risk of cancer.[103] On the other hand, high doses of intravenous synthetic vitamin C act as a drug in the body and may have therapeutic value in treating cancer.

How can I tell if my vitamin supplement is synthetic?

Read the label on the supplement bottle and see if the vitamin sources have the same names as those found in Table 8. If they do, they are synthetic.

Table 8. Common synthetic vitamins

Vitamin	Synthetic source listed as:
Vitamin C	Ascorbic acid
Beta carotene	Beta carotene (if source not given)
Vitamin B2	Riboflavin
Niacin	Niacin
Pantothenic acid	Calcium D-pantothenate
Folic acid	Pteroylglutamic acid
Vitamin D	Calciferol
Vitamin E	DL-alpha tocopherol, mixed tocopherols (unless plant-sourced)
Vitamin K	Menadione or phytonadione

Modified from: "How to Evaluate Vitamin and Mineral Products," Proevity CME. www.proevitycme.com

Most common synthetic vitamins have names ending in: hydrochloride, actetate, mononitrate, palmitate, menadione, phytonadione, and succinate.

MINERALS FROM ROCKS OR PLANTS?

Many of us are also deficient in minerals. All minerals come from the earth and eventually return to the earth. Minerals are classified as either inorganic or organic. Inorganic minerals in the soil are taken up by plants and changed into an organic form that our bodies can absorb and use more efficiently. For example, food-sourced magnesium is twenty-three times more soluble in the body than the inorganic crystal form of magnesium.[104]

Currently, most of the minerals found in supplements come from mined ores from the ground or they are produced synthetically in a lab. These mineral salts are not readily absorbed by the body; again, most of the pill is expelled from the body as waste. Pills have even been known to pass through the digestive system in tablet form, having never dissolved. Other forms of mineral supplements such as colloidal, chelated and ionic minerals all have limitations.[105] The ideal source of minerals comes from plants, but most plants contain only small amounts of minerals, so plant-sourced (organic) standardized mineral supplements in the past would have been a very large pill to swallow, because of its size. This is no longer the case as new technologies have emerged.

Are the minerals in your supplement inorganic or synthetic?

Many companies will claim that their product is better because they use a newfangled technology. Skip all the marketing hype and go straight to the label. If the nutrients are from inorganic or synthetic sources, then the supplement is really nothing new. If the supplement contains inorganic mineral salts or mineral/organic acid mixtures, they usually end in one of the following: ascorbate, aspartate, carbonate, chloride, citrate, gluconate, glycerophosphate, hydroxyapatite, iodide, lactate, malate, methionine, disulfide, orotate, oxide, dibasic phosphate, tribasic phosphate, picolonate, pyrophosphate, silicon dioxide, stearate, or sulfate.[106]

SUPER FOOD SUPPLEMENTS

A growing number of people are realizing the importance of food-form vitamins and minerals and as a result whole-food supplements have gained in popularity. Blends of super foods contain nutrient-rich foods such as greens, bee pollen, green tea, and wheat-germ oil. Other products are super juice blends, or fruit and vegetable extracts in capsules. This concept is taking hold because we know that nutrients found in real food provide greater health benefits.

The downside to these supplements is that they are not standardized, so the consumer has no idea what they are paying for. Unless independent tests are consistently done on the finished supplement, the consumer has no way of knowing the amounts of each nutrient in the supplement or whether nutrients are even present in the supplement. Standardization is a process used by supplement manufacturers to ensure that their products are consistent from batch-to-batch; it can provide some measure of quality control.[107]

It would be ideal if every plant was grown in perfect conditions, harvested and stored properly, and processed minimally. This would insure that the supplement contained high levels of nutrients. But in fact, consumers have no way of knowing exactly what they are buying unless the finished product has been tested for consistency of nutrient concentrations.

Several companies add synthetic vitamins and minerals to their *all natural* formula of fruit and vegetable extracts in order to reach the RDAs. This can be determined by reading the label and searching for synthetic and inorganic words mentioned above.

Juices: Buyer beware

Some juices sell for $20 to $30 a bottle. Independent studies have found that some of these juices contain fewer antioxidants than a bottle of grape juice off the supermarket shelf. I'm not implying that there is no value in any of these supplements, but buyers should read labels carefully and ask to view the results of independent lab tests done on the finished product.

Company reps often boast of amazing research done on their products, but you must look carefully at the research yourself to be sure that it was conducted on the finished product and is not just founded upon borrowed science. For example, a government study may find a very high antioxidant rating for vine-ripened blueberries. Many companies with blueberries in their product may simply take this research and apply it to their product. This antioxidant value holds true for the fresh, vine-ripened berry but may not be true for a processed juice.

STANDARDIZED PLANT SOURCED SUPPLEMENTS

This new standard of supplements includes those that contain standardized amounts of real food nutrients taken from plants. Real food dietary supplements provide natural, plant-based vitamins, minerals and phytochemicals that are standardized in amounts that meet daily recommended rates. Look for the words standardized, plant-sourced, and natural on the label. Then read the supplement facts on the label. The source should be from plants. If you find words from the list of synthetic vitamins and inorganic minerals on the label, this will tell you that these nutrients are synthetic or inorganic. When nutrients are plant-sourced, you will notice that the amounts per serving are much smaller. For vitamins, you will see units of micrograms (mcg) for plant sourced vs. milligrams (mg) for synthetic versions.

What to look for—NSF, NHP, and GMP designations

Make sure that the supplement you take is Natural Health Product (NHP) certified in Canada and National Sanitation Foundation (NSF) certified in the U.S. The supplement label should read NHP (if Canadian) or NSF (if American). This ensures that the product is safe, of high quality, and that there is a scientifically proven health benefit to taking the supplement. It is important to note that NHP and NSF certification does not indicate that a supplement is synthetic or plant-sourced. You will have to read the label to determine this. The manufacturer should also follow Good Manufacturing Practices (GMPs), which are guidelines that ensure a product has the identity, strength, composition, quality, and purity that it claims to have.

UNDERSTAND THE RESEARCH

If you would like to try a super-food blend of nutrients or a super juice, request to see the independent studies or tests conducted on the finished product(s). *Independent* means that the tests were done by a lab that doesn't have financial ties to the company. A quick review of the tests will show you if they were done on the food ingredients before they were processed or on the finished product itself. Make sure the research was conducted on the finished product by an independent lab. If there are no tests or studies, you could very well be wasting your money.

WHAT I HAVE DISCOVERED:

Consumer assumption:

"I really don't know much about supplements and don't need to because my chiropractor, nutritionist, naturopath, etc., is an expert. I can trust their recommendations."

You may choose to place all your faith in one expert, but you may not be satisfied with the results. I don't believe that any one expert has all the answers.

An expert may recommend a specific line of supplements because he or she sincerely believes it is the best for you, but even the expert may be sincerely wrong. I once had a discussion with a nutritionist about supplements. We agreed about the importance and benefits of taking natural, plant-derived vitamin/mineral supplements as opposed to synthetic versions. When she informed me that she carried an all-natural line of vitamins and minerals, I took a bottle from her shelf, read the label, and commented that the nutrients in the supplement were synthetic. She replied, "Well, there's synthetic and then there's synthetic." Bottom line: she had invested in this particular line of products and believed that they were cutting edge even though they were synthetic. Here was a nutritionist with a university degree in nutrition who should have known better, yet she was more intent on selling a particular line of supplements in which she had invested substantial time and money, despite the synthetic content. I was initially shocked but quickly recalled that I have experienced this attitude with other health-care providers in the past.

Supplements are big business, and unfortunately many health care professionals are predominantly educated about supplements by supplement company representatives.

Lesson Learned

You must take responsibility for your health. You cannot leave your health solely in the hands of any so-called expert. This is why you must have a basic understanding of dietary supplements so that you will know what will benefit your health and what is simply a waste of money. Use common sense, your intuition, and your gut instincts. If you feel something isn't good for you, get a second opinion. If a supplement makes you feel sick, stop taking it and ask questions.

SUPPLEMENTATION IN A NUTSHELL:

1. Regularly eat whole-food meals which include many servings of vegetables and fruit each day. The USDA recommends 7–13 servings of produce each day, depending on your size and age. Be sure to vary the types and colors of produce you eat. Buy local when available and certified organic if possible.
2. Make sure the supplement company follows GMPs and that the supplements are NSF (in the U.S.) or NHP (in Canada) certified.
3. Read labels! If a company uses the phrase *all natural*, don't believe it until you read the ingredients label yourself. What are the sources of the vitamins and minerals? The source of the nutrient determines if your body will absorb it, not whether it is in liquid form or some other method of delivery. The body is designed to receive most nutrients from plants.
4. If you would like to try a super-food blend of nutrients, or a super juice, request to see the independent studies or tests conducted

on the finished product(s). Independent means that the tests were done by a lab that doesn't have financial ties to the company. A quick review of the tests will show you if they were done on the food ingredients before they were processed or upon the finished product. Make sure the research was conducted on the finished product by an independent lab. If there are no tests or studies, you could very well be wasting your money.

5. You will experience the greatest benefits to your health if you include standardized natural plant-based vitamins, minerals, antioxidants, phytosterols, phytonutrients, glyconutrients, and essential fatty acids.

Taking the right supplements is an important part of a wellness plan. It is valuable to have a basic understanding about the different types of supplements available on the market. This knowledge will save you time and money. Also, as an informed consumer you will know which questions to ask. Basic principles go a long way.

FINDING IT DIFFICULT TO REACH YOUR IDEAL BODY SHAPE?

Have you been dieting for years only to put the weight back on after each diet? For more than 20 years, North Americans have been on a low fat diet, and yet today obesity is epidemic. Some experts blame our sedentary lifestyle. Large amounts of the wrong fats in our diet and a lack of activity are two factors that can play a role in obesity, but these alone cannot account for the epidemic that we face today. I believe that we are missing three very important factors—specifically nutritional deficiencies, dysbiosis of the digestive tract (an imbalance in the microbes found in the GI tract), and our increased consumption of processed carbohydrates and simple sugars.

In this chapter we have discussed the importance of optimal nutrition in the structure and function of our cells, tissues and organs, and body systems which regulate our appetite, mood, blood sugar levels and metabolism. Many clients have stated that as their nutrition intake was optimized through a whole food eating plan and taking in plant-sourced nutritional supplements, they experienced more energy, a greater sense of well-being and fewer cravings.

Once again, nutrition is the foundation of wellness—including weight management.

The Role of Gut Microflora in Obesity

The types of microbes (bacteria, yeasts, parasites, etc.) that live in the GI tract can impact our general health in many ways, including the development of obesity and insulin resistance.[108] The importance of maintaining health-promoting microbes in the GI tract will be discussed in greater detail in the chapter titled, Minimize Silent Infections (page 85).

It is important to mention that a growing body of evidence suggests that the types of microbes that live in the GI tract may play a role in obesity as they are "an important environmental factor that affects energy harvest from the diet and energy storage in the host."[109]

How Processed Carbs Turn into Fat

Processed carbohydrates such as white flour and white rice are starchy carbs that have been stripped of their natural fiber and nutrients during processing. They may be fortified with a few synthetic vitamins, but as discussed in the Synthetic Vitamins section of the book (page 73), synthetic nutrients do not provide the same benefit to the body as plant-sourced nutrients. Furthermore, all the nutrients that were once present in the original whole food are not added back into the processed food, even if in a synthetic form.

The glycemic index (GI) ranks carbs from 0–100 according to the degree that blood sugar levels rise after the carb is eaten.[110] Processed carbs are digested by the body and absorbed into the blood stream more quickly than complex carbohydrates, resulting in a rapid rise in blood sugar and higher insulin levels. Processed carbs will have a higher GI rating. They provide a burst of energy, followed by a drop or crash in energy. If our blood sugar levels increase higher than what our body needs, some of the extra sugar will be stored as glycogen in the liver and muscles, and the rest will be changed into fat and stored in fat cells.[111]

In contrast, complex carbohydrates contain natural fiber which slows down digestion resulting in a gradual rise in blood sugar and insulin levels.[112] These carbs have a low GI rating. Eating complex carbs gives us a more stable energy supply for a longer period of time which makes us feel satisfied (not hungry) for longer.

We replaced fat with sugar

As we accepted recommendations to reduce saturated and total fats in our diet, the food industry decreased the fat content in processed foods, but then added simple sugars to these foods to make them tastier. Simple sugars end in *ose* and include glucose, galactose, fructose, sucrose, and maltose. Some of the most common sources of simple sugars are baked goods and desserts, jellies, candy, processed cereals, dairy desserts and milk products, fruit drinks and soft drinks.[113] According to the U.S. Department of Agriculture's Economic Research Service, the consumption of sugars and sweeteners increased in the country by 19% between the years 1970 and 2005.[114]

When we substituted simple sugars for the fat in processed foods, we not only nullified any benefit of reducing bad fat in weight management but actually made matters worse. Dr. Robert Lustig, pediatric neuroendocrinologist at the University of California, San Francisco, explains that excess sugar consumption "drives fat storage and makes the brain think that it is hungry, setting up a vicious cycle."[115] Also, sugar (sucrose) has been shown to have addictive properties and has an effect on the brain similarly to certain drugs that are often abused.[116]

A growing number of researchers and clinicians are concerned that excessive amounts of fructose from high fructose corn syrup (HFCS) is a greater concern in obesity than sucrose. HFCS was first introduced into our processed foods about 40 years ago because it is more cost effective than sucrose. It is the sweetener found in most soft drinks and other processed foods. Each person in the U.S. consumes on average 60 lbs of HFCS per year.[117]

Results from a study at Princeton University found that "all sweeteners are not equal when it comes to weight gain."[118] These studies found that lab animals that were fed HFCS had a significantly higher weight gain than lab animals fed sucrose (table sugar). It is interesting to note that the overall caloric intake was the same for both groups.[119]

Furthermore, a six month study found that lab animals with a normal diet and access to HFCS gained 48% more weight than animals fed a normal diet without access to HFCS. The lab animals with access to HFCS showed symptoms of the human metabolic syndrome with increased triglycerides and higher concentrations of belly fat.[120]

HFCS is either 42% or 55% fructose and the balance is mostly glucose. Sucrose is made up of one molecule of glucose and one molecule of fructose. The noted difference in weight gain in the lab animals may be partially due to the different ratios of sugars found in the HFCS and sucrose sweetener, but is more likely due to the fact that the fructose in HFCS is free and not bonded to the glucose molecules.[121]

No digestion is required when free fructose is eaten. It can be absorbed and used immediately by the body. Sucrose molecules found in cane sugar or beet sugar have one molecule of fructose bonded to one molecule of glucose. This bond must be broken or digested by an enzyme before the fructose and glucose can be absorbed into the body.

Also, studies have shown that consuming large amounts of fructose in the diet results in lower levels of the appetite suppressing hormone leptin, which is important in the regulation of blood sugar levels.[122] Leptin signals to the brain that the body has had enough to eat, producing a feeling of being satisfied.

What's worse—sugar or HFCS?

"High-fructose corn syrup and sucrose are exactly the same," says Dr. Lustig, "They're equally bad. They're both poison in high doses."[123] Dr. Lustig believes that sugar is more harmful to our health than fat.

Consumption of either sugar or HFCS leads to higher levels of artery clogging fats made by the liver and deposited in the arteries. Fructose from HFCS adds a greater insult as it also damages the liver and structural proteins, and fuels excessive consumption of calories.[124]

Stop Dieting

Focus less on weight loss and more on wellness. As you build your Four Pillars of Wellness, I am confident that your energy levels, health, mood, and the ability to release fat will all improve. Added bonuses include a decrease in food cravings and an increase in the body's ability to eliminate toxins as fat is burned. This supports a stable, permanent move toward your ideal body shape.

> **Q. Which nutrient is the most important?**
> **A. The one you are most deficient in.**

As we build the first pillar of wellness, *Optimizing Nutrition*, we are supporting the body to operate at its peak, and to repair and heal itself when necessary. Optimizing nutrition alone can add many quality years to our lives.

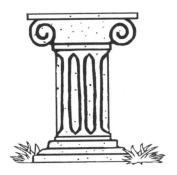

Pillar #2
Minimize Silent Infections

This may be the most important section of the book because minimizing silent infections and dysbiosis is the component of wellness that most people are not aware of. Once you you truly understand the concepts covered here, sickness will no longer be a mystery and the fear associated with disease will be dispelled. I say *really understand* because this will require you to embrace a philosophy that is not widely accepted by the conventional medical model. This new philosophy works, makes sense, and is cost effective. It is not a new concept, it is a return to the basics which have been forgotten for some time. Our current health care philosophy is the product of large industries that make more money when disease is a mystery and health care is a complicated process requiring literally hundreds of costly treatments and medications that must be taken for life.

From the moment we are born until the moment we die, the world of microbes is trying to *take us out*. This is just a fact of life and it's called war. The war is between our immune system and the microbes that are trying to take over our bodies and recycle us before we are ready to go. This battle is constant and can take place in various parts of our body simultaneously. Most often we aren't even aware that these wars are occurring.

By restoring, supporting and protecting our body's natural defenses, which includes the normal flora (good bacteria found on the skin and in mucous membranes—GI tract, sinuses, genitourinary) and our immune system, we are able to keep bad microbes from taking over, which in turn will add many quality years to our life.

WHAT ARE "SILENT INFECTIONS?"

Silent infection is probably a new term for most people. Silent infections are chronic or slow-growing infections in the body that lack the normal clinical signs of an acute infection. Because they lack the traditional symptoms of infection, the medical community has largely dismissed the notion that they exist and cause disease.

When we think of an infection we think of a flu, fever, headache, sore throat, cough, runny nose, redness or pus in an infected area. These are typical clinical signs that alert our doctor that we have an infection. The medical community believes that human pathogens cause illness through infection and that infection must be displayed through the typical clinical symptoms described above. If you do not display these symptoms, they cannot determine that you have an infection. Thus the belief that a chronic, low grade infection can cause disease has largely been dismissed by our medical community.

Despite the medical community's view on this, a growing body of science supports the belief that silent infections can and do cause inflammation and disease in the body even though they do not display the typical clinical symptoms of infection. Researchers at the Mayo Clinic found that nearly 70% of participants who suffer with arthritis were carriers of "clinically silent infections."[125] Another study published in the *Annuals of Rheumatic Diseases*, found that if proper tests were conducted, the researchers were able to determine the causative pathogen (bad microbe) in 56% of arthritis patients.[126] These patients suffered with gastrointestinal or genitourinary dysbiosis.

Researchers at St. George's Hospital Medical School in London, detected Mycobacterium paratuberculosis (MAP) in 92% of patients suffering with Crohn's disease.[127] And finally, the first manifestation of the autoimmune disease polyendocrinopathy-candidiasis-ectodermal dystrophy (APECED) is Candidiasis, an overgrowth of the yeast Candida.[128]

Thus, research concurs that microbes such as yeast/fungi, bacteria and many other parasites directly cause health issues, inflammation and disease in people and do not always display typical clinical symptoms associated with infection.

COULD INFLAMMATION BE CAUSED BY INFECTION?

Inflammation is the body's natural protective response against disease-causing microbes, damaged cells, and other harmful agents. Inflammation is a common symptom in disease. The medical community can measure the level of inflammation in the body, but for the most part, cannot explain what is causing the inflammation in disease. With mounting evidence supporting the notion that silent infections and dysbiosis exist and cause disease, many experts are asking the question "could inflammation be caused by infection?"

According to Dr. Alex Vasquez,[129] there are now at least fourteen different methods that microbes use to cause immune dysfunction and inflammation in the body without causing a typical infection.

There are many reasons why microbes create very different immune responses in humans: the severity of the infection, the types of toxins and other metabolites produced by the microbes, the deficiencies that the infection creates in its host, and the biochemical and genetic individuality of the person are just a few.

THE GI TRACT: YOUR LIFELINE TO HEALTH

While this may sound like the wild-wild west, this section will give you a new appreciation for your digestive tract (GI tract). Your GI tract starts at the mouth and includes all organs between the mouth and anus, but for the purpose of this book I will focus on the large and small intestines. Along the GI tract, nutrients are extracted from our food and absorbed into the bloodstream to provide raw materials for the body to build and fuel healthy cells. A healthy GI tract is essential for vibrant health. Many people unfortunately have less than healthy GI tracts, and therefore less than optimal health.

A healthy GI tract is a marvel. It is not only the place where digestion and absorption of our food occurs, but it also houses about 70% of our immune system. The actual surface area of the GI tract is close to the size of a football field. This large area is needed for the body to absorb all the nutrients we require to keep our bodies healthy and strong.

The GI tract is our lifeline to health. This is a happening place. Here most nutrients are extracted from foods, while some are produced by good bacteria. The nutrients are then transported into the blood stream to feed our cells. Wastes from the body return to the GI tract and are removed from the body. If the GI tract is healthy, it will deliver nutrients to build healthy cells, tissues, and organs and glands. If the fuel is lacking due to a poor diet or a sick GI tract, you won't experience optimal health.

If you have suffered tummy troubles for some time then you will definitely want to focus on restoring health to this area. The more you restore balance, the better you will feel. It is helpful to work with a health care provider who understands dysbiosis and knows how to help you restore balance.

The human body is made up of approximately 100 trillion cells, yet the number of microbes living in the GI tract is approximately 10 times that number.[130] This vast area in the GI tract should be mostly populated by good or friendly bacteria. These are the good guys. You may be familiar with the good bacteria acidophilus which is found in fresh yogurt. You may have also heard the word probiotic which is another name for the good guys. There are many strains of good bacteria that help us to digest and absorb our food, make nutrients for us, and keep the bad guys (yeasts, bad bacteria, and other parasites) from overpopulating our GI tract. In a healthy digestive system, the bad guys are present in minute numbers compared to the good guys. The dense population of good guys in the GI tract competes for food and space, and prevents the bad guys from increasing in numbers and making us sick.

OFF TO A ROUGH START—DYSBIOSIS IN INFANTS

The GI tract of a fetus is sterile. As the child is born it passes through the birth canal where ideally, the baby is introduced to the good bacteria. The good guys establish themselves in the infant's digestive system, creating a healthy environment that promotes proper digestion and absorption of nutrients, and also providing nutrients for the infant.

Unfortunately, if the expectant mom has had yeast infections in the past (before pregnancy), the change in hormones during pregnancy can cause a flare-up of the vaginal yeast infection.[131] As a result, the infant passing through a birth canal can be literally coated with yeast. This can be the start of dysbiosis in the child's GI tract (this will be discussed further in Section Three—Women's Health Issues starting on page 194.)

Remember, dysbiosis is a fancy word for disharmony in the digestive tract. Basically, the microbes that live in the digestive tract are out of balance. The good or friendly bacteria that should be present in great numbers have been reduced, while the population of bad bugs (yeasts and other parasites) is too great in number. If these bad guys thrive in our body, they will produce toxins, rob us of important nutrients, and cause inflammation which affects our ability to absorb nutrients.

A few days after birth, the mom may notice that her child becomes increasingly fussy and later on colicky as the child experiences abdominal discomfort caused by gas produced by the yeast overgrowth. At this point, the mom doesn't know what the child wants so she just keeps feeding the child in a desperate hope to settle the baby. The child may develop a significant case of cradle cap[132] and later may develop oral thrush, persistent diaper rashes that are only remedied by an antifungal cream, and recurrent bladder or ear infections.

It is typical for breastfed babies to have more than one bowel movement each day, but a breastfed child with dysbiosis may not have a bowel movement for several days. The child may also experience anemia as the established yeast robs the child of iron.[133] This can be a rocky start for both the child and mom, and is an example of how dysbiosis can start even before antibiotics have been introduced.

How do I know all this? Unfortunately it comes from personal experience.

THE PANDORA'S BOX OF HEALTH CARE

In my view, the overuse of antibiotics is a Pandora's box that has destroyed the delicate balance of flora (good bacteria) in the human GI tract and consequently is one of the biggest—if not the biggest—contributor to chronic disease.

Antibiotics definitely serve a purpose. If someone is dying from pneumonia or any other acute bacterial infection then yes, a course of antibiotics is warranted. Antibiotics have saved many lives, but for years they have been used excessively. The consequence of this is finally becoming apparent.

In coaching hundreds of people in wellness over the past 10 years, I have found that dysbiosis is epidemic, and I believe that the biggest culprit in this tragedy is the overuse of antibiotics. Our highly processed North American diet certainly adds fuel to this fire, but it all starts with the destruction of the delicate balance and natural defenses that sustain health.

This disaster was not created intentionally, but it is a grave tragedy nonetheless. The vast majority of health care professionals did not understand just how serious and wide spread the consequences of frequent and long-term antibiotic use would be.

There is no longer an excuse for any person to ignore the mounting research that supports the fact that our digestive health has been seriously compromised by the overuse of antibiotics. It is vital that this information becomes evident to health care professionals and the general public so that we can reverse the upward trend of chronic disease and prevent many others from suffering needlessly.

How it all starts

It is important to note that commonly prescribed broad spectrum antibiotics kill the targeted bacterial infections but have no effect on yeast and fungi, nor many other parasites found in the GI tract.

When a child or adult takes a broad spectrum antibiotic, the targeted bacterial infection is eradicated, but the friendly bacteria in the gut are also destroyed, leaving an open field for less desirable microbes such as yeast and other fungi, and parasites to flourish. The bad guys now have lots of room to grow and are quite happy with our high glycemic North American diet that is rich in simple sugars.

Fungi, yeasts and many other microbes love sugar. Eating highly processed carbohydrates (white carbs and simple sugars) fuels the infection; our blood sugar rises quickly and feeds the bad guys.

If you have ever made bread you will remember that adding sugar to the yeast causes the mixture to bubble or ferment as gas is produced. Fermentation also occurs in our GI tract when we suffer with bacterial and/or yeast/fungal overgrowth and eat generous amounts of processed carbohydrates.

This is how dysbiosis starts for many people. The first symptoms of dysbiosis in the GI tract are discomfort, pain, gas, bloating, constipation, and/or diarrhea... similar to many of the symptoms of inflammatory bowel disease.

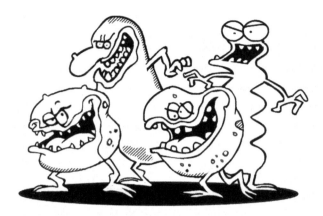

The Bad Guys—bacteria, fungi and other parasites

Why pick on Candida?

The medical community has focused on bacteria and viruses as the cause of disease, yet there are many other parasites that also cause disease. Candida albicans is the most important human fungal pathogen because it frequently causes infections of the mucous membrane and can be a life-threatening systemic disease.[134] Yeasts and other fungi, mycobacteria, plasmodia, mycoplasma, flukes, and worms, are just some examples of the many parasites that can be involved in human disease.

It is extremely frustrating that the majority of the medical and scientific communities refuse to even consider that yeasts and other fungi can cause disease in healthy individuals. Most doctors believe that yeast/fungi are just nuisances and are only a health concern in immunosuppressed individuals who are undergoing cancer treatments, organ transplants, and other clinical treatments and procedures. They also believe that yeast/fungi only cause annoying symptoms such as dandruff, vaginal infections in women, jock itch in men, and fingernail or toenail fungal infections. For some reason they seem to refuse to even question the role of fungi in disease.

It is accepted by the medical and scientific community that common side effects of antibiotics include stomach upset, diarrhea and vaginal yeast infections in women.[135] The Merck Manuals Medical Online Library states "Antibiotics taken by mouth tend to kill the bacteria that normally live in the vagina and prevent yeast from growing. Thus, using antibiotics increases the risk of developing a yeast infection."[136] If this is true, then what about the GI tract? This same scenario occurs in the gut, but for some reason we are told that the immune system will deal with it and that good bacteria will repopulate on its own.[137] This sounds great in theory, but how do the experts come to this conclusion? If medicine and science is based on empirical evidence, then where is the research that supports such claims? Any woman suffering with vaginal yeast overgrowth or a person with toenail fungus or dandruff knows first-hand that the infection will not go away without treatment.

Secondly, how can we be certain that the GI tract (which is close to the size of a football field) will repopulate with good bacteria on its own and quickly enough to discourage the growth of the bad guys?

The typical North American diet which includes an abundance of processed carbs and simple sugars will support the growth of the existing bad guys and will not promote the re-growth of the good guys.

This book will highlight research that supports what many of us have known for years. Candida and other fungi are very often intimately linked with chronic disease—even in people that were not originally immunosuppressed, and yeast/fungal overgrowth actually causes disease for many people. Chronic yeast/fungi infections are epidemic in North America and totally overlooked by the majority of our medical and scientific community.

FUNGAL INFECTIONS

Yeasts and other fungi are the recyclers of the world. If they ever became extinct, we would have heaps of dead organic matter all around us. Fungi are found everywhere and although about 70,000 species have been identified, the true number of members is estimated to be 1.5 million. In the past 20 years clinicians have observed a growing number of fungal infections and approximately 20 new infectious fungal species appearing annually.[138]

Why is there such an increase in fungal infections? Some experts believe that this is the result of an increase in immune-suppressed patients that are dealing with viruses, leukemia, organ transplants, and more intensive and aggressive medical practices.[139]

Disease trends are on the rise and as a result there are more immuno-suppressed patients, but I would argue that the marked increase in disease is a direct product of the overuse of antibiotics which we know leads to fungal overgrowth.

I will refer to Candida often because it is a well-known, extremely hardy human pathogen and is normally found in small numbers in the GI tract of a healthy person. Candida is a type of yeast and a member of the kingdom Fungi. We don't have to go to a foreign country to be infected with Candida. Nearly 20 Candida species have been identified as being associated with human infections.[140]

Candida lives in several forms in the GI tract. The first form is the non-disease-causing single-cell form. This form is present in small amounts in a healthy GI tract and doesn't cause harm. It basically gets a free ride by eating some of our food, but its population is not abundant enough to make us sick.

If the good guys are wiped out as a result of antibiotics, the harmless form of Candida morphs into the disease-causing filamentous form, which generates discomfort (dysbiosis symptoms) in the GI tract.

The filamentous form is similar in shape to a strong root system which can penetrate tissues in the body. As Candida continues to prosper in the GI tract, its root-like branches push through the walls of the GI tract into the blood stream. Leaky gut results as the infection directly damages the lining of the GI tract causing it to become more permeable, thus allowing bigger molecules of food and other substances (toxins, microbes) to enter the blood stream that normally would not. Causes of this condition include Candida, and other infectious agents as well as non-steroidal anti-inflammatory drugs, and ethanol.[141]

The walls of a healthy GI tract normally act as a barrier and will only allow specific substances to cross into the bloodstream. Leaky gut is linked with allergy and autoimmune disease.[142] It is believed that this condition causes food sensitivities as the immune system becomes hypersensitive to the inadequately digested proteins and other foods substances that enter the bloodstream.[143] The immune system will defend the body and attack these large foreign molecules that should not be present in the blood stream.

Candida then migrates to different parts of the body and further infects and penetrates other tissues. Candida infections can occur in any part of the body including the meninges (the system of membranes that envelopes the central nervous system), heart valves, brain, lungs, liver, eyes, spleen, and kidneys.[144]

Because yeast is a common inhabitant of the human digestive tract it will often show up in test results even in healthy people and is therefore not considered a health risk. Also, fungal overgrowth is usually a slow, chronic process which develops over years[145] without the typical clinical symptoms of an acute infection, which means that most doctors do not recognize it as a health concern. Finally, tests for determining fungal overgrowth are often inconclusive and difficult to access. Again, this is because the medical community does not believe that yeast overgrowth poses a health risk.

Why is it so difficult to treat fungal infections?

There are several reasons why it is challenging to permanently eradicate yeast overgrowth:

1. Yeasts love sugar, and our North American diet feeds the infection. While treating a yeast infection, it is vital to avoid all processed carbs and simple sugars and eat limited amounts of certain complex carbohydrates to avoid major fluctuations in blood sugar levels. Yet, even when this recommendation is followed, the body will maintain a healthy blood sugar level which Candida will still benefit from. Candida in the bloodstream is very sensitive to blood glucose levels.

Blood glucose concentrations increase Candida's resistance to our immune system and to treatments by antifungal medication.[146]

2. The GI tract is a warm, moist, and nutrient rich environment which provides ideal growing conditions for yeast and other parasites.

3. Trying to repopulate the GI tract with good guys is challenging. As probiotic supplements are taken or homemade yogurt that contains probiotics is eaten, many of the good guys are destroyed by stomach acid and digestive juices, but some will survive. Remember that the combined surface area of the small and large intestine is about the size of a football field. Antibiotics are able to destroy much of the good guys within a week or two, and at this time we do not have therapies or technologies that are able to restore the good guys as quickly as they are destroyed. It is wise to take a high potency effective probiotic after a course of antibiotics as some of the good guys will survive the journey through the acidic stomach.

4. Within a short period of time, yeast/fungi will form biofilms which are difficult to treat. Biofilms are a protective coating which prevents medications and probiotics from reaching the yeast/fungi.

5. Fungi are hard to treat because they have various life forms and, over time, penetrate deep into our tissue.

6. Yeasts are very adaptive to antifungal treatment; they become resistant to a particular treatment quite quickly.

7. High stress, lack of sleep, a sedentary lifestyle, lack of sunshine, certain medications, fluctuations in hormones and a diet that is rich in processed carbs all encourage fungal overgrowth.

How yeast/fungus can make us feel sick and lousy

We are just beginning to understand how and why fungal infections make us feel lousy:

- Yeast/fungal overgrowth can rob us of important nutrients like glyconutrients, B vitamins, and iron,[147] causing nutritional deficiencies.
- Yeasts and bad bacteria can produce molecules that interfere with

normal metabolism in the body. Many of these molecules are observed in higher levels in patients with migraines, depression, weakness, confusion, schizophrenia, agitation, and arthritis.[148]

- Neurotoxins in the gut from yeasts and bacteria may contribute to autistic symptoms.[149]
- Candida can affect immune function by producing toxins that suppress the immune system (see Table 10 page 176).
- Yeast directly weakens our immune system by producing enzymes that digest our antibodies which we require to fight infection. These same enzymes can also destroy keratin and collagen leaving us more vulnerable to infection by other bad microbes and antigens, which can lead to allergy (see Table 10 page 176).[150]
- Women with chronic vaginal infections are nearly two times more likely to develop allergic rhinitis or hay fever[151] and people with chronic yeast overgrowth are more likely to suffer with allergies.[152]

It has been my experience that when fungal overgrowth is controlled, immune function improves, and autoimmune, inflammation and allergy symptoms subside.

Why am I sensitive to gluten?

Gluten is a protein found in wheat, barley, oats and rye. It is also present in smaller amounts in the ancient grains kamut and spelt. In celiac disease (CD) the lining of the small intestine becomes inflamed and damaged which hinders the absorption of nutrients from food. Over time, people with CD run the risk of becoming malnourished. Inflammation occurs as the immune system becomes sensitive to gluten and produces antibodies against gluten. For some scientifically unknown reason, the immune system treats gluten as a foreign invader and therefore will attack and destroy it.

Celiac disease must be taken seriously and treated appropriately as it increases the risk of:[153]

- Other autoimmune disorders
- Bone diseases (fractures, osteoporosis, and abnormal curvature of the spine)
- Anemia
- Hypoglycemia
- Certain intestinal cancers
- Infertility or repeated miscarriage
- Liver disease

Doctors diagnose celiac disease though symptoms and a blood test. Many people who are sensitive to gluten have come to realize that gluten makes them sick so they choose to avoid eating it. The immune system will only produce antibodies against gluten when it is eaten in the diet. Therefore, if you are sensitive to gluten and avoid it, you will likely get a false negative test result. If you want a fairly accurate test result, you must eat gluten on a regular basis before you are tested for CD. Although CD is known to affect about 1% of the population, this number is an underestimate because not all doctors inform their patients that they must be eating gluten regularly before the test, and because the blood test itself is not 100% accurate. CD is mainly undiagnosed with a ratio of twenty undiagnosed individuals for every diagnosed individual in the U.S.[154]

People with yeast overgrowth are most often sensitive to gluten[155] and therefore gluten must be avoided during the Initial Phase of the Candida treatment program.

> The HWP1 Candida protein contains many identical sequences of amino acids as the gliadin proteins found in gluten.

Why does the immune system become sensitive to gluten? Although there is no widely accepted answer for this, researchers in the Netherlands[156] have uncovered a clue that may help explain why the immune system turns against this seemingly harmless protein complex: gliadins are the part of gluten that celiacs become sensitive to.

Candida uses the protein HWP1 to attach to the lining of the GI tract. This protein helps the yeast become established and cause infection. Proteins are made up of amino acids. These researchers have discovered that the HWP1 Candida protein contains many identical sequences of amino acids as the gliadin proteins found in gluten.[157]

Thus the immune system may attack the gliadin proteins of gluten as though they were part of the Candida overgrowth. This group of scientists believe that Candida albicans is a trigger in the onset of CD.[158]

> This group of scientists believe that Candida albicans is a trigger in the onset of CD.

If a gluten free diet has been followed for several months while yeast overgrowth is treated and symptoms of CD persist, visit your health care provider. Sometimes other parasites or bacterial overgrowth in the small intestines may hinder the relief of symptoms.[159] In fact, one study found that most celiacs with persistent symptoms had small intestine bacterial overgrowth.[160]

It doesn't make sense that such a complex immune system would act chaotically and attack gluten for no reason. What is interfering with the immune system's ability to function optimally? Why is it creating such a strong response to something that is harmless? The presence of a silent infection would be a more logical explanation for this phenomenon and a growing body of research is supporting this belief.

If inflammation in CD is the product of our immune system fighting infection and we treat CD by merely taking a pharmaceutical that suppresses our immune system, we may experience temporary symptom relief from the inflammation as the immune system is down regulated by the drug; but in the long run the infection is still there and will continue to gain ground in the body and negatively affect our health in many other ways as seen in the list on pages 112-114.

MY JOURNEY WITH DYSBIOSIS

...has been the worst and, in the end, one of the best experiences of my life. For years this journey was very frustrating. My motivation and desire in telling my story is that it will inspire health care professionals to understand that fungal infections and dysbiosis are not just a nuisance or a consequence of immune suppressed patients, but that they are epidemic; they can directly suppress the immune system and they are a direct cause of disease. I also hope that others will gain a better understanding of what they are going through and see that they are not alone in their suffering.

It is so important to pay attention to the small warning signs our body gives us before big health issues develop; it is so much easier to maintain or improve health before disease sets in.

> It is so important to pay attention to the small warning signs our body gives us before big health issues develop.

Dysbiosis started for me at birth. My mom had suffered a history of undiagnosed stomach complaints and allergies, so I was one of those unfortunate babies coated with more of the bad guys than good guys during birth. I now believe that I was heavily infected with yeast at birth.

As a result, I was extremely constipated as a baby even though I was breast fed. Our family doctor recommended that my mom should eat a chocolate bar each day to relieve my constipation. While it did resolve the issue, it definitely didn't promote health.

At the age of about 18 months I was anemic, even though I received iron-enriched rice cereal as well as many fruits, vegetables and meat. My mom avoided feeding me all grains except rice because I didn't tolerate the gluten cereals.

Could it be that the anemia I experienced as a young child was a direct consequence of the Candida infection I picked up at birth? Candida requires iron to live, and research shows that it has the ability to extract iron from its host. It possesses iron-acquisition proteins on its surface that can extract iron from hemoglobin, transferrin, lactoferrin and ferritin.[161]

I grew up in a small farming community in Southern Alberta, Canada. Whenever I was sick with a high fever, a sore throat or cough, our family physician would prescribe antibiotics. He never ordered a test to see if the infection was caused by a virus or bacteria. I suffered with constipation, frequent stomach aches and swollen eyes throughout my childhood. I was very slim and people would always comment "You are so skinny," which made me very self-conscious.

By age 12, my stomach aches had become a concern so my doctor decided to remove my appendix. After the surgery he reported that my appendix was healthy. This unnecessary surgery was very unfortunate because I lost a my appendix which plays an important role in immune function and I was left with a large scar.

As I entered my teens, the stomach aches and constipation continued and to add to this, a bad case of acne. Once again my doctor had the solution. This time he recommended that I take the antibiotic tetracycline for several months. I followed his advice because he was the expert and I hated the acne. The acne did settle down but my tummy troubles continued.

Now fast forward to my first years of marriage. At the age of 21 I was expecting my first child. The experts recommended that I drink at least 4 glasses of milk a day, so I did just that and more. As a result, I experienced a lot of gas pains during the night, especially during my third trimester. I would get up in the middle of the night and walk around because of the discomfort.

My daughter was born a healthy almost nine-pound baby. I nursed her for the first nine months of her life. Within a few months, she developed a diaper rash that wouldn't settle down. The doctor prescribed an antifungal ointment that cleared up the rash. This rash would occasionally reappear but was kept in control with the antifungal ointment.

Within a few months my daughter developed thrush, which is a Candida infection in the mouth. I used the prescribed antifungal drops for her mouth and disinfected all her toys, but still couldn't get rid of this infection. The doctor finally prescribed gentian violet, which is a bitter, purple medication similar to iodine. I painted the inside of her mouth with this medication for the recommended length of time. She absolutely hated it and would gag and throw up each time I applied it.

Even after using gentian violet, the thrush would return. I was at my wit's end and was referred to a pediatrician who asked me if I was feeding my daughter yogurt. I replied yes and said that I had heard that yogurt would discourage yeast infections. She explained that in her experience, when parents stopped giving their children yogurt, the thrush would settle down.

You are probably wondering how this could be possible, given what we have learned about the good bacteria found in yogurt. The problem was that I was feeding my daughter the fruit and sugar sweetened yogurt from the grocery store. This yogurt contained very little (if any) good bacteria and ample sugar which fed the yeast. At that time, I knew very little about Candida. I did stop giving her the yogurt which resolved the issue.

When my daughter was about 15 months old I became pregnant with my son. I almost lost him in the first trimester when I began to hemorrhage. I was confined to bed rest for several weeks, and the bleeding settled down by the fourth month. During this pregnancy, I experienced chronic fatigue, which I dismissed as being part of pregnancy and being a mom. I felt run down; like I was coming down with a flu, although I never did get the flu. Later in the pregnancy I told my doctor that I would get a tingle running down my arm when I bent my neck. He though it was unusual but dismissed it. Once again I drank lots of milk during my pregnancy.

My son arrived four weeks early, and at birth, he quickly turned blue. At first the specialists thought that it was his heart but soon determined that he had premature lung disease. My son required 10 days of oxygen in an incubator. Fortunately he recovered very quickly and didn't require a ventilator.

Within a couple of weeks at home he became fussy. I had to watch the foods I ate because certain foods made him colicky. He developed the same diaper rashes his sister had experienced, and once again I controlled them with an antifungal cream. He thrived as I nursed him.

As my son approached six months of age I began to suffer with insomnia and continued chronic fatigue. I was severely sleep-deprived because of the insomnia, but just carried on with my busy life.

One warm sunny afternoon, my husband, children and I visited a local park. I noticed a black spot in the center of the vision in my left eye. I kept rubbing my eye but it wouldn't go away. By the second day the spot had grown significantly. I was concerned and made an appointment to see an eye specialist. The specialist informed me that I had optic neuritis (inflammation of the optic nerve). By the third day I had lost all vision in my left eye. It was as if a black patch was placed over the eye. I also had a terrible headache and debilitating fatigue. I made another trip to the eye specialist and was given a prescription for prednisone. He informed me that severe optic neuritis was often an indicator of multiple sclerosis (MS) and thus referred me a neurologist at a local university multiple sclerosis clinic to receive a proper diagnosis.

> By the third day I had lost all vision in my left eye.

The neurologist confirmed the diagnosis of MS. My symptoms were: extreme fatigue, headaches, severe optic neuritis, and tingling and weakness in my legs. The neurologist informed me that in time I would become totally disabled. He warned me about people who would try to sell me *snake oil* products that would promise a cure and insisted that there was absolutely nothing that would change the fact that I would become completely disabled either quickly or slowly.

Shortly thereafter, my mother-in-law sent me the book, *The Yeast Connection*, by Dr. William Crook. As I read the book, I found that I related to many symptoms Dr. Crook described. I scored very high on the Candida survey and, for the first time since my diagnosis, felt that there might be hope that I would once again enjoy quality of life if I dealt with the yeast overgrowth.

All my Candida symptoms stemmed from my GI tract—or so I

thought—because I had never been treated for vaginal yeast infections in the past. I began to learn about a nutritional program called the Candida diet and started to implement the necessary changes. I noticed that I felt better as I avoided gluten grains, sugar, and processed carbs.

Whereas some experts believe MS might be caused by a virus, it didn't make sense to me because viruses are not alive; they don't eat food, and I found that my digestive and MS symptoms worsened when I ate more carbohydrates. I came to believe that, for me, the cause of the MS and digestive condition had to be something that benefited from carbs... for example yeast or bacteria.

My doctor prescribed the antifungal drug Nystatin. I continued to research and read everything I could find on health and wellness, and Candida in particular, including Dr. William Truss' book, *The Missing Diagnosis*, as well as Jeanne Marie Martin and Dr. Zoltan Rona's book *The Complete Candida Yeast Guidebook* and Dr. Luc Schepper's book *Candida*. These medical doctors all echoed the same message that I was starting to very seriously believe: that Candida was intimately linked to my disease, and that it might even be the direct cause of the MS. The more I read, the more excited and hopeful I became.

> These medical doctors all echoed the same message that I was starting to very seriously believe: that Candida was intimately linked to my disease, and that it might even be the direct cause of the MS.

When I was placed on prednisone for the optic neuritis, I had to quit nursing my son immediately. I had a healthy breastfed baby for the first six months of his life—as I avoided the foods that he didn't tolerate. He was never sick and had healthy weight gain despite being born prematurely. I started him on a dairy-based formula and within a short period of time he began to develop frequent respiratory infections. In his preschool years he developed allergies, asthma, eczema, and an anaphylactic reaction to peanuts. I took him off all dairy and gluten products, and limited all refined carbohydrates as was recommended by the doctors who wrote the Candida books. His eczema subsided and his asthma improved so much that he would only have to use an asthma puffer once or twice each winter when he developed a persistent respiratory infection that settled in his lungs.

I continued to work on improving my own wellness. Over the next eight years, I tried many natural therapies and supplements with the goal of eradicating the yeast from my body and building up my immune system. I tried acupuncture, Chinese medicine, iridology, reflexology, allergy testing and desensitization, chiropractic care, oxygen therapies, and safe nutritional supplements and herbs. I also had my amalgam (mercury) fillings replaced and did chelation. I spent thousands of dollars on complementary and alternative medical (CAM) therapies. Some therapies and supplements helped while others did nothing. The only consistency I found was that the more I worked at killing the yeast overgrowth, the better I felt.

All my hard work was paying off. I was able to keep the MS in remission for eight years without the use of any pharmaceuticals beyond the original prednisone, which I used for a few weeks during the initial attack. I really felt that I had the Candida under control. My energy was back and I felt great. I decided to go back to school and start my science degree. My husband and I wanted more children, so after 8 years of debating with myself as to whether my body would handle it or not, we decided to have another child.

The third pregnancy went well—no hemorrhaging. I had lots of energy and was able to finish my semester at university just before delivering my son. During pregnancy, I continued on the Candida diet, avoiding dairy, gluten and processed carbohydrates. I ate healthy, with lots of vegetables, some fruit, raw nuts, meats, millet and brown rice. I avoided caffeine. As the labor started, my doctor checked to see how far along I was and informed me that I had quite a yeast infection. I was horrified! How could this be? I didn't experience any of the typical symptoms of a vaginal yeast infection and I had just spent 8 years eradicating the yeast from my body. My doctor mentioned that yeast overgrowth is common during pregnancy. The yeast infection was so bad that after delivery I thought I had a bladder infection. The test came back negative and the doctors said that it was just the yeast infection. More on this subject in Section Three—Women's Health Issues found on page 194.

I delivered a healthy nine-pound baby boy who was coated in yeast during birth. My son became fussy within a day and then developed colic. He was breastfed and should have had two to three bowel movements each day, but he had them only once every week or two. For the first two months of his life he cried and fussed most of the night and my fatigue and insomnia returned. I had him checked by a pediatrician who said he couldn't find anything unusual and felt he was a perfectly healthy child.

Because of my history with Candida, I suspected that my son might be suffering with dysbiosis caused by yeast overgrowth so I visited a naturopath. The naturopath confirmed this and gave me a homeopathic Candida remedy. This remedy, together with probiotics, settled his colic and within a month we were both sleeping through the night.

But this wasn't the end of our Candida problems. After nursing my son for several months, I started having issues with nursing: plugged milk ducts to be exact. I will discuss this further in the Women's Health Issues section. After trying many remedies and antibiotics, my last resort was to either quit nursing or try the antifungal drug Fluconazole. This drug resolved the issue and I was able to continue nursing.

Over the next few years I continued to have problems with Candida. Once again I suffered tummy troubles and oral thrush. Occasionally I would experience a slight tingling in my legs, a definite warning sign. I worried that I might run out of complementary treatments and therapies that would keep the Candida from taking over my health. I followed the Candida diet, and rotated many antifungal treatments, both herbal and pharmaceutical, with not as much success as the first time. This may have been due to the fact that I was under a lot of stress finishing my science degree and raising a young family. Also, I was ten years older. The antifungal treatments kept the yeast from taking over my body but I had to continually rotate them as the yeast would adapt to the various treatments.

Regardless of how alkaline my diet was, my pH was always acidic. It was always below seven, and the worse I felt, the lower my pH was. I did take another prescription of the antifungal Fluconazole for three weeks. It is interesting to note that after taking this antifungal, my pH finally jumped above seven and stayed there for months. It is well documented that yeast and bacteria produce acids. Candida albicans is able to acidify its environment when glucose is present, which allows production of a protein enzyme which in turn makes the yeast more virulent.[162,163]

> It is well documented that yeast and bacteria produce acids.

Could the acids produced by the yeast overgrowth have caused the low pH? And as the yeast overgrowth was knocked back by the drug, less acid was produced and thus my pH increased?

It is important to note that my medical doctor performed comprehensive blood work on me several times and the test results always came back in the normal range. I was a perfectly healthy person plagued with yeast overgrowth.

In the year 2000 I was introduced to glyconutrients. At that time I had just finished my science degree and found the science of glycobiology fascinating. Although my degree was in biology and I had completed a full year of biochemistry, I had never been introduced to them.

As previously discussed on page 66, glyconutrients support optimal cellular communication (how our immune cells interact with our tissue) and immune function. I felt that this support would be beneficial because with MS and autoimmune in general, there is a miscommunication between the immune cells and other cells of the body. Also, with the recurrent Candida infections, immune support would definitely be helpful.

Therefore, I decided to start taking this supplement and noticed a significant improvement to my health. I had more energy and a greater sense of well-being. Also, my immune system was better able to keep the yeast under control after taking this supplement. I have now taken glyconutrients for more than ten years and can sincerely say that they are the last supplement that I would ever give up.

But why did glyconutrients help me? Was the marked improvement that I experienced after taking this nutrient simply the result of correcting a nutritional deficiency caused by the yeast overgrowth? For me, that seemed to be the most reasonable answer.

It is well known that yeast cell walls contain mannan, and that mannan is part of the glyconutrient mannose. Could correcting a simple nutritional deficiency be one of the main reasons why so many of us have experienced such improvements to our health after supplementing with this class of nutrients? There is no widely accepted answer to this issue and clearly more research is needed.

Yeast overgrowth will benefit from some of the nutrients provided by supplements. The goal is to provide the body with enough nutrition from whole foods and supplements so that nutrient deficiencies are corrected. This will enable the body to fight the silent infection more successfully.

I have not found a miracle cure that will eliminate yeast overgrowth once and for all. I have had the most success in reducing the yeast population and regaining balance by discovering, building and upholding The Four Pillars of Wellness. These four pillars have allowed me to enjoy an amazing quality of life.

Diagnosing fungal overgrowth?

This next section is for educational purposes. It is not a substitute for the care of a health care professional. If you suffer with a serious medical condition, it is important to work with your doctor or other health care professional.

The information here will help you determine if you are dealing with chronic yeast/fungal overgrowth. Experts believe that at least 80% of the population deals with some degree of fungal overgrowth because of the combination of overusing antibiotics and our high-glycemic diet. I believe that the percentage of people with fungal overgrowth is much higher than 80%. Whatever the percentage, it is clearly an epidemic. I will share the most successful ways that I have found to treat yeast overgrowth and silent infections so that you can have long term success.

What you learn here will help you take responsibility for your health. You will be well-equipped to ask the right questions when looking for and working with a health care professional. If your medical doctor won't work with you, then find one who will, or look for a good naturopathic doctor. Pharmacists can also be a great help as many of them are knowledgeable about pharmaceuticals, supplements and herbal remedies.

RULING OUT CANDIDA

If you suspect that you are dealing with a silent infection (an infection that the doctors cannot find), the first microbe to rule out is Candida, because it is the most common yeast that can make us very sick.

Systematic yeast overgrowth has been associated with at least 80 potential symptoms.[164] Doctors believe that a specific disease will exhibit a specific set of symptoms in all people affected by that disease. It's no wonder why doctors have such a hard time believing that yeast/fungi overgrowth could display such a diverse list of symptoms and diseases in people.

Physicians also resist accepting the idea that chronic fungal overgrowth can cause disease because current tests for fungal infections are very poor and chronic fungal overgrowth doesn't display the typical symptoms of an acute infection. When you visit your doctor with a sore throat, swollen glands and a high fever, it is clear to your doctor that you are dealing with a typical acute infection. Your doctor will take a swab of your throat and the lab will determine what type of microbe is making you sick. When you walk into your doctor's office with a bunch of unrelated vague symptoms, he or she will have no idea where to start. If your doctor has no experience in treating silent infections, it would be like looking for a needle in a haystack. For the most part, a doctor's medical training has not taken into consideration the idea that yeast or fungus could possibly cause disease in healthy people, but rather only in immune suppressed individuals.

There are many reasons why we see such an array of symptoms in people with fungal infections. Some include differences in gender, environment, in the type of fungal pathogen present, and the fact that each one of us is genetically and biochemically unique.

Many experts believe that symptom surveys are very helpful in diagnosing yeast overgrowth. The more symptoms you check off on the survey, the greater the likelihood that you suffer with yeast overgrowth.

Although surveys are helpful, I believe the most valuable tool in diagnosing yeast overgrowth is a careful consideration of a person's medical history. It has been my experience that the number and types of symptoms vary widely among people. For example, a small child may suffer with recurrent ear infections, a teenager may have irritable bowel and severe acne, while a 50-year-old may complain of five or more symptoms from the list on page 112.

Just one yes answer could mean that you have yeast/fungal overgrowth:

_____ 1. Have I used antibiotics in the past?

_____ 2. Have I been on a cortisone-type medication or blood pressure medication in the past?

_____ 3. For females—have I used the birth control pill or hormone replacement therapy?

_____ 4. Does my mother currently or in the past (before I was born) show symptoms from the list on page 112? Did my mom take antibiotics in the years before I was born?

_____ 5. Do I suffer with one or more of the symptoms from the list on page 112?

From personal experience coaching others in wellness, the more yes answers in your response, the more likely you have suffered with chronic yeast or fungal overgrowth for some time. I have observed that even one yes can indicate yeast overgrowth.

Other diagnostic aids

Other diagnostic tests for yeast overgrowth include stool samples as well as antibody and organic acids tests. Unfortunately lab tests can be difficult to access and false positive and negative test results are common.

Stool tests for Candida are not very reliable. Candida is normally found in the GI tract so test results may not be accurate. The stool test may be more beneficial when checking for other parasites that may hinder improvements. As mentioned earlier, other parasites can become established if a person has suffered with yeast overgrowth for a long period of time.

A promising stool analysis test that measures the presence of DNA from various good and bad bacteria, yeast and parasites found in the GI tract is available. This test avoids the limitation of trying to keep the microbes alive while transporting the stool sample to the lab. It also measures microbes that only live in the absence of oxygen. This test can be ordered by a health care professional.

The Radioimmunoassay and the Enzyme-Linked Immunosorbent Assay (ELISA) tests have been reported to be useful in measuring Candida antigen and antibody levels in the blood. Both are available in the U.S. but not in Canada.

The Urine Organic Acids Test (OAT) is a valuable test that provides a health care professional with a snapshot of a patient's overall state of health. It measures levels of molecules that are by-products of the activities of our cells and the digestion of our food. They also measure dysbiosis by detecting elevated concentrations of waste products produced by the bad guys. This lab test provides a broad range of information and can also be ordered by a health care professional.

The Candida Saliva Test is a self-test that can be done at home. I haven't included it because I am skeptical about its accuracy. There are many factors that can affect saliva. However, if you wish to try this self-test you will find the directions on the Internet.

It has been my experience that some naturopathic doctors rely too heavily on the Vega machine to diagnose or dismiss yeast overgrowth. A Vega machine is an electronic acupuncture instrument used to diagnose allergies, illness, and many other health issues in the body. I realize that this instrument may be useful in confirming or supporting the findings of other tests but I don't believe that results from the Vega instrument should carry more weight than a patient's history and symptoms. I have several clients who in the past demonstrated numerous characteristic symptoms of chronic yeast overgrowth, but the Vega machine showed that their yeast levels were not a concern. If this is your experience you may want to get another opinion.

The best diagnostic approach is to use a person's history, lab test and survey results, and to undertake a trial period of following the Candida program.

THE SURVEY

Common Symptoms of Chronic Yeast Overgrowth

General Symptoms:
- Craving for and overeating sweets, breads and/or alcohol

Digestive System Symptoms:
- Bloating
- Gas
- Cramps
- Diarrhea or constipation
- Alternating between diarrhea and constipation
- Sensitive to dairy or gluten
- Heart burn
- Belching

Nervous System:

- Abnormal fatigue
- Spaciness
- Anxiety
- Depression
- Poor memory
- Tingling
- Burning
- Weakness
- Joint pain or swelling
- Lethargy
- Brain fog
- Mood swings
- Insomnia
- Confusion
- Numbness
- Muscle Aches
- Paralysis

Skin Symptoms:

- Dry or irritated lips
- Rash, blisters or rough skin on the inside of the cheeks of the mouth. You may bite the inside of your lips.
- Hives
- Allergies
- Swollen or puffy eyes — may be worse in the mornings
- Sensitive to chemicals or molds
- Eczema
- Psoriasis
- Acne
- Fungal finger or toe nail Infections
- Ring worm
- Athlete's foot

Endocrine System Symptoms:

- Hypo or hyperthyroidism
- Adrenal fatigue

Recurrent Infection Symptoms:

- Recurrent infections of the ear, sinuses, bladder, or throat

Female Symptoms:

- Recurrent vaginal infections
- Occasional white cottage cheese-like vaginal discharge
- Lumpy breasts, cysts
- Plugged milk ducts while nursing
- Premenstrual syndrome (PMS)—depression, mood swings, bloating, fluid retention, cramps, craving for sweets, headaches prior to menstruation
- Low sex drive

Female Symptoms (continued):

- Menopausal symptoms
- Vaginal itch, or burning
- Heavy bleeding during menstruation
- Cramping during menstruation
- Endometriosis

Male Symptoms:

- Jock itch
- Prostatitis
- Impotence
- Genital Rash
- Chronic rectal or anal itch
- Low sex drive

Candidiasis is associated with almost every medical condition:

- Joint pain
- Itchy burning eyes
- Spots or lines in vision
- Inability to gain weight
- Iron deficiency (anemia), or low ferritin
- Autoimmune disease
- Cancer
- Recurrent infections
- Chronic sinusitis
- Hypoglycemia
- Eating disorders
- Alcoholism
- Addictions
- Autism, hyperactivity, learning disabilities in children can be manifestations of fungal overgrowth

*List compiled from:
1. Complete Candida Yeast Guidebook by Jeanne Marie Martin with Dr. Zolton Rona
2. Staying Healthy with Nutrition by Dr. Elison M Haas
3. The Yeast Connection Cookbook by Dr. William Crook
4. Suzie Cohen—Dear Pharmacist http://dearpharmacist.com/?p=1346

YOUR GAME PLAN TO COMBAT THE ENEMY

When I say *combat the enemy*, I am referring to knocking the population of fungus in the body back so much that it no longer causes unpleasant or disease symptoms. I have been researching this topic for over twenty years and to this day I have not met one person who has found a complete, permanent cure. To me a cure means that the problem and resulting symptoms are gone permanently and that you never have to worry about it again.

It doesn't work like that with yeasts and fungi in general. The longer you have had an imbalance of fungal overgrowth in your body, the more established the yeast biofilms and root network will be in your tissues.

Fungi are around us. They are in the air we breathe, the water we drink and the food we eat. We cannot avoid being in contact with fungi. As I mentioned earlier, fungi are one of the great recyclers of organic matter. There is a constant tug-of-war between microbes which are trying to take over our body and literally decompose us— earlier than we would like—and our immune system, which is actively fighting them off and defending our body. If we work at keeping our immune system strong and the population of bad guys down to a minimum in our body, we will experience a better quality of life and a longer life. It really is that simple!

Four steps to combat the yeast/fungal enemy:

1. Starve the enemy
2. Kill the enemy
3. Reestablish the good guys
4. Surveillance

Steps 1, 2 and 3 are done simultaneously

1. STARVE THE ENEMY

This is the most important part of the game plan. It entails an eating plan that does not encourage the growth of yeast and other bad microbes. The goal is to eat just enough complex carbohydrates (carbs) to maintain your health but not enough to encourage fungal growth. Since yeast and fungus love simple sugars it is vital that you avoid all processed carbohydrates (anything white—white rice, white flour and pasta, all sugar, and white potatoes) and avoid many starchy complex carbohydrates such as gluten grains and most fruit for the short term. Most dairy products are also avoided for the short term.

Excess carbohydrates are a feast for yeast. Our body will maintain a healthy blood sugar level so that our brain is able to function. The yeast will still feed on sugar in our blood, but if we restrict the amount and type of complex carb for the short term, less carbs will be available for the yeast to feed on in the GI tract. Also, as we eat limited amounts of specific complex carbs, we avoid spikes in our blood sugar levels that result from eating simple sugars, processed carbs and even large amounts of complex carbs. A large serving of a low glycemic complex carb will cause blood sugar levels to reach a higher than normal peak, and it will take a longer period of time for blood sugar levels to return back to normal.[165] Remember, if you suffer with yeast overgrowth and binge on carbs, the yeast will binge right along with you!

Children

Children are resilient and most recover from dysbiosis quickly by eating a whole food eating plan, avoiding dairy, gluten and sugar, taking nutritional supplements and supplementing with an effective probiotic.

The Initial Phase of the Candida eating plan is a healthy plan. Children with suspected fungal overgrowth should not limit complex carbs as their bodies are actively growing. A child's body will usually respond much quicker than an adult. See the children's section on page 139.

Pregnant women and nursing mothers

Pregnant or nursing moms should not follow the strictest part of this eating plan as it limits simple sugars which the baby needs for development. If you are pregnant or nursing you should eliminate all processed carbs and eat a whole food eating plan (whole grains, lots of vegetables, some fruit, good quality protein, nuts, good fats, etc.). If you suspect that you have Candida overgrowth during pregnancy, you can still follow a gluten free, dairy free, and processed carb free eating plan. If you do not tolerate dairy products, make sure to take a good quality calcium supplement. Always work with an experienced health care professional.

Kidney disease or other serious illness

If you suffer with kidney disease or any other serious medical condition always let your doctor know what you would like to do with respect to diet and supplements. The anti-Candida eating plan tends to be higher in protein, which may prove difficult for people with kidney disease.

There are many versions of the anti-Candida eating plan in books and on the Internet. Some are accurate and others are not. If you are inexperienced, it may seem confusing. The goal is to follow a plan that will deliver positive results as quickly as possible. The eating plan is a very important part of the program. If you don't follow it, your success will be very limited.

Some anti-Candida eating plans recommend avoiding all starchy carbs (including non-gluten whole grains such as brown rice, quinoa, millet, buckwheat, etc.) for a short period of time, while other programs will allow you to eat modest amounts of these complex carbs. If you choose the plan to omit all starchy carbs for a short period of time, you will lose weight. If you have a physically demanding job, you may choose to eat four or five meals during the day instead of just three meals. Snacking on the right foods is fine. Just listen to your body and eat when you are hungry.

I have found that the anti-Candida eating plan as suggested by Doug Kaufmann, and the plan designed by Jeanne Marie Martin and Dr. Zoltan Rona, are two very reliable approaches to the problem. Doug Kaufmann is a veteran in the war against Candida. For many years he has been preaching the message that fungal overgrowth can cause poor health.

I bought the first edition of *The Complete Candida Yeast Guidebook* in 1996. I am grateful that Dr. Rona stepped out and shared his experience and knowledge and I'm sure that he dealt with his share of criticism from his peers. He is a true hero. There are other pioneers in this field and because of these individuals, I have been able to live a full, vibrant life for the past 20 some years.

> ## Two excellent resources for the Candida eating plan:
>
> 1. *The Complete Candida Yeast Guidebook 2nd Ed.* by Jeanne Marie Martin with Zoltan Rona MD
> 2. *Eating Your Way to Good Health* by Doug Kaufmann knowthecause.com

The following is a plan to give you direction on how to get started. It includes a list of which foods to avoid and which foods to enjoy as well as helpful tips that I have learned over the years. I haven't included many recipes because once you learn which foods to avoid you will be able to take many of your favourite healthy recipes and modify them to fit the plan. You can also find recipes in the two books that I recommended or simply go online. Just make sure that the recipe meets the following criteria and plan your meals ahead.

PREP PHASE: DURATION: 1–2 WEEKS OR LONGER IF NECESSARY

These two weeks will ease you into the program. Think of this as a time of preparation; a time to clean up your diet so that the Candida diet won't be such a drastic change. If you normally eat a lot of processed foods, you may need the full two weeks to prepare. If you need more than two weeks, take it. If you have already made healthy changes to your eating plan you may only need one week to prepare—you be the judge.

During this time it is important to become familiar with the Initial Phase of the Candida program. Create a menu plan that includes foods and recipes that you enjoy and that discourage fungal growth. A big key to your success is being prepared. If you are starving, unprepared and not sure what to eat, chances are you will grab food that will set you back.

If you are accustomed to eating processed foods, the Prep Phase should be time you spend preparing more meals from scratch using whole foods. You will notice that the foods you can enjoy in the Prep Phase are foods that are close to their original or natural state. Preparing meals doesn't have to be time consuming. It just takes planning ahead.

During the Prep Phase you will also want to ensure that you are taking high quality, plant-sourced nutritional supplements to fill in the gaps of what is missing from our food.

BASIC GUIDELINES:

Avoid These Foods

- Processed carbohydrates — (anything white) white flour, white rice, white pasta, white sugar

- Processed meats (sandwich meats, sausage, bacon, ham, etc.)

- The sweeter fruits (oranges, apricots, cherries, bananas, melons, plums, grapes, mangoes, pineapples, exotic fruit and dried fruit)

- Fruit that is over or under ripe

- Caffeine (coffee, tea), alcohol, pop, sodas and juices

- Baked whole grains which include yeast

- Dairy products except plain yogurt and real butter
  Note: You can get your daily recommended intake of calcium from whole foods, veggies, nuts, seeds and a good calcium supplement.

- All sweeteners (natural and artificial).

- White, navy, lima, haricots, northern, pea beans

Prep Phase—Enjoy These Foods

Whole grains
- Eat one serving of a whole grain with each meal.
- Best Choice—brown rice, quinoa, millet, buckwheat—old fashioned oat flakes, steel cut oats, brown pot barley (if you tolerate gluten)
- Second Choice—100% whole grain products made without yeast (only if you tolerate gluten).

Fruit
- Eat one serving of fruit each day—preferably in the morning, on its own at least 15-30 min. before a meal.
- Best choice—apple (organic), berries (organic), kiwi, avocado, white grapefruit, fresh lemon juice, fresh lime juice, fresh papaya.

Meats—chicken, turkey, beef, lamb, and pork
1. Best choice—organic, grass fed (beef)
2. Second choice—hormone free, antibiotic free, not fed animal byproducts
3. Third choice—lean conventional meat

Seafood
1. Best choice—wild fish
2. Second choice—farmed fish

 *Certain chemicals (like mercury and PCBs) are concentrated in certain types of fish. If you eat a variety of fish you are less likely to load up on one chemical. The Environmental Defense Fund website outlines which fish should be avoided and how many times a month you can safely eat each type of fish.
 Visit: http://www.edf.org/page.cfm?tagID=17694*

Whole Natural Eggs
1. Best choice—organic, free range, organic fed or vegetarian fed
2. Second choice—buy local and free range if possible.
3. Third choice—conventional

Tofu (cooked only), Beans (cooked only), and Legumes
- Adzuki (aduki, azuki) cooked only
- Black beans
- Chick Peas
- Fava beans

- Kidney beans
- Lentils (red, green, brown and gray)
- Mung beans (dry or sprouted)
- Pinto Beans
- Red beans
- Romano beans

Nuts

- All nuts are okay except peanuts, pistachios and walnuts (if no allergies)
1. Best Choice—Buy bags of fresh whole nuts and store in the freezer. Take out what you will eat each day.
2. Second best—dry or oven roasted, no added salt

Soya nuts aren't really nuts. Avoid eating soya regularly (fermented soya is okay if tolerated—tofu, miso, etc.). Research indicates that eating soya regularly may impair the absorption of minerals.[166]

Dairy Products

- Choose—Plain yogurt and real butter. Some people tolerate plain yogurt and others do not. If you are not sure, avoid it until you have completed the first two phases of the program. Then reintroduce it and you will know if it works for you or not.
1. Best choice—Homemade yogurt from organic milk (incubate for 24 hrs.). This is loaded with good bacteria.
2. Second choice—Buy organic plain yogurt. Open up one or two capsules of probiotics (the good bacteria) and mix into the yogurt.
3. Third choice—Buy plain yogurt and mix probiotic capsules in it.

Vegetables

- All vegetables except corn, mushrooms, & potatoes
1. Best Choice—local certified organic
2. Second best—local, little or no pesticides
3. Third choice—organic but not local (looks healthy)
4. Fourth choice—conventional produce
- Organic produce can be expensive and isn't always available.
- *The Environmental Working Group's Shopper's Guide to Pesticides* recommends eating produce from the Dirty Dozen list only if it is organic and choose non-organic from the Clean Fifteen group if necessary. By doing so you will dramatically lower the pesticide load in your tissues.

Shopper's Guide to Pesticides

The Dirty Dozen (Highest Pesticide Load)	The Clean Fifteen (Lowest Pesticide Load)
Celery	Onions
Peaches*	Avocado
Strawberries	Corn*
Apples*	Pineapples*
Blueberries	Mangoes*
Nectarines (Imported)*	Sweet Peas
Sweet Bell Peppers	Asparagus
Spinach	Kiwi
Lettuce	Cabbage
Kale/Collard Greens	Eggplant
Potatoes*	Cantaloupe*
Grapes (Imported)*	Watermelon*
	Grapefruits
	Mushrooms*
	Sweet Potato*

Dirty Dozen & Clean Fifteen modified from the Environmental Working Group's Shopper's Guide to Pesticides *www.ewg.org*
* To be avoided during the Prep and Initial Phases of the Candida program

Drinks
• Purified water
• Caffeine free herbal teas (hot or cold —organic is best)
• If socializing—sparking water or club soda (beware of the extra salt in club soda) with fresh squeezed lemon, lime, or mint leaves.

Good Fats
• Include good fats from real butter, and virgin olive, grape, flax or coconut oils—choose cold-pressed not hydrogenated

For sweeteners see the Initial Phase page 128.

Modified from: *Eating Your Way to Good Health* by Doug Kaufmann; *Fuller Healthy Groceries* by Lauren Fuller; *The Allergy and Asthma Cure* by Dr. Fred Pescatore; *The Complete Candida Yeast Guidebook* by Jeanne Marie Martin with Dr. Rona.

Helpful Hints:

- Remember to always listen to your body. If something doesn't agree with you, stop, re-evaluate, and get advice from an experienced health care professional.
- At least 50% of your plate or meal should be made up of a variety of non-starchy vegetables.
- Include a variety of raw veggies or slightly steamed veggies.
- If you suffer with any inflammatory bowel condition you may want to steam vegetables until your health improves. Avoid vegetables that bother you at this point.
- Make enough for dinner so that you have leftovers for lunch or dinner the next day. Refrigerate leftovers.
- Prepare your lunch the night before. Pack leftovers from dinner in glass, stainless steel, or ceramic—not plastic.
- Be creative with recipes—use fresh or dried herbs (not irradiated).

Snacks

1. Carrot, celery and other veggie sticks dipped in nut butter (almond butter, tahini, filbert butter, etc.)
2. Nuts and seeds (almonds, pecans, cashews, sunflower seeds, pumpkin seeds, filberts, sesame seeds)—if no allergies
3. One serving of fruit from the above list each day
4. Leftovers—home-made soups, stews, stir-fries, etc.
5. An occasional (no more than one or two each day) whole grain rice cake (not the bleached white kind), with nut butter on it
6. A salad—throw nuts on top. Salad dressing—apple cider vinegar, fresh lemon juice or fresh lime juice with olive oil, flax seed oil or grape seed oil (oils should be cold pressed or virgin)

When you are comfortable with the food choices of the Prep Phase of the program and have researched and planned for the Initial Phase of the program it is time to move on to the next step—The Initial Phase.

INITIAL PHASE: DURATION: 1–4 MONTHS OR AS LONG AS NECESSARY

The Initial Phase eating plan of the Candida program, together with therapeutic agents (see Kill the Enemy section page 143), provides the most effective treatment for yeast overgrowth at this time. The more strictly the eating plan is followed the more quickly improvements will be enjoyed. Although this eating plan may scare some of you at first, you will find that, as you quickly become accustomed to the changes in your food choices, you will thoroughly enjoy the improved energy and greater sense of well-being. Many of you that have dieted for years will appreciate that you won't have to starve yourself while on this program. You will be able to snack on the appropriate foods when necessary.

Avoid These Foods

- Processed carbohydrates—(anything white) white flour, white rice, white pasta, white sugar

- All gluten grains: wheat, barley, oats, rye, kamut, spelt, etc.

- Processed meats (sandwich meats, sausage, bacon, ham, etc.)

- The sweeter fruits (oranges, apricots, cherries, bananas, melons, plums, grapes, mangoes, pineapples, exotic fruit and dried fruit)

- Fruit that is over or under ripe

- Caffeine (coffee, tea), alcohol, pop, sodas and juices

- Baked whole grains which include yeast

- Dairy products except plain yogurt and real butter
  Note: You can get your daily recommended intake of calcium from whole foods, veggies, nuts, seeds and a good calcium supplement.

- All sweeteners (natural and artificial).

- White, navy, lima, haricots, northern, pea beans

The Initial Phase of the eating plan is very similar to the Prep Phase. In the Initial Phase all gluten grains are avoided and the types of fruit are more restricted. It is important to continue taking high quality plant sourced nutritional supplements to fill in the gaps of what is missing from our food.

Initial Phase—Enjoy These Foods!

Whole grains
- If you can afford to lose weight, avoid all grains (wheat, barley, rice, millet, quinoa, buckwheat, rye, oats, corn, etc.) for the first two weeks. After two weeks add a modest serving of brown rice, wild rice (not the sweet varieties), millet, quinoa, and buckwheat to each meal.
- If you are slim and cannot afford to lose weight, eat one small whole grain serving of brown rice, quinoa, millet or buckwheat with each meal.
- *Avoid all gluten grains for the first month or more—until all your digestive complaints have stopped for some time. Then re-introduce 100% grains (yeast free) and monitor how you feel. If symptoms return, it is too soon to add this grain back into your eating plan.*

Fruit
- Eat one serving of fruit each day—preferably in the morning, on its own at least 15-30 min. before a meal.
- Best choice—green apple (organic), berries (organic), kiwi, avocado, white grapefruit, fresh lemon juice, fresh lime juice, fresh papaya.

Meats—chicken, turkey, beef, lamb, and pork
1. Best choice—organic, grass fed (beef)
2. Second choice—hormone free, antibiotic free, not fed animal byproducts
3. Third choice—lean conventional meat

Seafood
1. Best choice—wild fish
2. Second choice—farmed fish
* Certain chemicals (like mercury and PCBs) are concentrated in certain types of fish. If you eat a variety of fish you are less likely to load up on one chemical. The Environmental Defense Fund website outlines which fish should be avoided and how many times a month you can safely eat each type of fish. Visit: http://www.edf.org/page.cfm?tagID=17694

Whole Natural Eggs

1. Best choice—organic, free range, organic fed or vegetarian fed
2. Second choice—buy local and free range if possible.
3. Third choice—conventional

Tofu (cooked only), Beans (cooked only), and Legumes

- Adzuki (aduki, azuki) cooked only
- Black beans
- Chick Peas
- Fava beans
- Kidney beans
- Lentils (red, green, brown and gray)
- Mung beans (dry or sprouted)
- Pinto Beans
- Red beans
- Romano beans

Nuts

- All nuts are okay except peanuts, pistachios and walnuts (if no allergies)
1. Best Choice—Buy bags of fresh whole nuts and store in the freezer. Take out what you will eat each day.
2. Second best—dry or oven roasted, no added salt

  *Soya nuts aren't really nuts. Avoid eating soya regularly (fermented soya is okay if tolerated—tofu, miso, etc.). Research indicates that eating soya regularly may impair the absorption of minerals.[167]

Vegetables

- All vegetables except corn, mushrooms, & potatoes
1. Best Choice—local certified organic
2. Second best—local, little or no pesticides
3. Third choice—organic but not local (looks healthy)
4. Fourth choice—conventional produce
- Organic produce can be expensive and isn't always available.
- *The Environmental Working Group's Shopper's Guide to Pesticides* recommends eating produce from the Dirty Dozen list only if it is organic and choose non-organic from the Clean Fifteen group if necessary. By doing so you will dramatically lower the pesticide load in your tissues.

Shopper's Guide to Pesticides

The Dirty Dozen (Highest Pesticide Load)	The Clean Fifteen (Lowest Pesticide Load)
Celery	Onions
Peaches*	Avocado
Strawberries	Corn*
Apples*	Pineapples*
Blueberries	Mangoes*
Nectarines (Imported)*	Sweet Peas
Sweet Bell Peppers	Asparagus
Spinach	Kiwi
Lettuce	Cabbage
Kale/Collard Greens	Eggplant
Potatoes*	Cantaloupe*
Grapes (Imported)*	Watermelon*
	Grapefruits
	Mushrooms*
	Sweet Potato*

Dirty Dozen & Clean Fifteen modified from the Environmental Working Group's Shopper's Guide to Pesticides *www.ewg.org*
 * To be avoided during the Prep and Initial Phases of the Candida program

Dairy Products

- Choose—Plain yogurt and real butter. Some people tolerate plain yogurt and others do not. If you are not sure, avoid it until you have completed the first two phases of the program. Then reintroduce it and you will know if it works for you or not.
1. Best choice—Homemade yogurt from organic milk (incubate for 24 hrs.). This is loaded with good bacteria.
2. Second choice—Buy organic plain yogurt. Open up one or two capsules of probiotics (the good bacteria) and mix into the yogurt.
3. Third choice—Buy plain yogurt and mix probiotic capsules in it.

Drinks
- Purified water
- Herbal teas (organic is best)—caffeine free
- If socializing—sparking water or club soda (beware of the extra salt in club soda) with fresh squeezed lemon, lime, or mint leaves

Good Fats
- Include good fats from real butter, and virgin olive, grape, flax or coconut oils—choose cold-pressed not hydrogenated

Sweeteners
- The natural sweeteners stevia and xylitol do not feed yeast and can be used sparingly. Large amounts of xylitol can cause diarrhea and thus should be avoided.

Modified from: *Eating Your Way to Good Health* by Doug Kaufmann; *Fuller Healthy Groceries* by Lauren Fuller; *The Allergy and Asthma Cure* by Dr. Pescatore; *The Complete Candida Yeast Guidebook* by Jeanne Marie Martin with Dr. Rona.

Tips for Eating out

Many restaurants are beginning to offer healthier choices but you will still have to make modifications. Here are some tips:

- Let your server know that you have health issues and that you must avoid certain foods. They are usually very accommodating.
- When ordering salads, request no dressing on your salad and ask for a slice of lemon or lime and some olive oil on the side instead.
- Choose meat that is grilled and not breaded or marinated. Tell the server that you can have butter, oil, salt, pepper, garlic, and herbs—but no sauces.
- Many restaurants will let you substitute the French fries for a salad or vegetable.

Initial Phase Breakfast Ideas

Fruit: one serving per day, 1 green apple (if tolerated—if it gives you gas—avoid it), berries, ½ grapefruit, V8 Juice. Eat fruit at least 30 min. before breakfast.

Or fresh squeezed lemon or lime in water—drink during the day or upon arising before breakfast.

1. Omelets (2-4 eggs + splash of water + salt and pepper to taste)
   - Mediterranean: add spinach, fresh basil, canned plain olives, green onions, tomatoes
   - Mexican: cook with coconut oil. Add onions, peppers, avocado (at end), tomatoes, cilantro, chilli powder, paprika, cumin

2. Baked green apple + cinnamon + raw ground nuts + home-made yogurt. Or baked apple slices + cinnamon topped with ground nut flour and drizzle with butter

3. Fried eggs + stir fried veggies: onions, peppers, bok choy, ginger, etc.

4. Vegetable frittata: 6 eggs, 1 cup broccoli flowerets (steamed until tender), 1 red pepper, 1 onion, butter, 1/3 cup yogurt (optional), finely grated lemon rind, pinch oregano, pinch rosemary, sea salt. Sauté onion and pepper. Beat eggs, add yogurt, mix in veggies. Add butter to pan and pour mixture into pan. Cover and cook about 5 min. until underside is golden.

5. Poached eggs

6. Zucchini muffins
   3 cups nut flour (almond, pecan)
   2 tsp. cinnamon
   1 tsp. baking soda
   ½ tsp. salt
   3 eggs, beaten
   3 cups grated zucchini
   1/3 cup melted butter

   Optional:
   - During the Initial Phase the natural sweetener stevia can be used Caution: stevia is about 100 times sweeter than sugar so use sparingly
   - During the Surveillance Phase, use smashed banana or small amount of raw honey as sweeteners

- Mix almond flour, cinnamon, salt and baking soda in a bowl. In a separate bowl beat eggs, add melted butter, and zucchini. Mix liquid mixture with dry mixture. Bake in muffin tins lined with papers at 350° F (180°C) for about 20 min. or until done. Freeze extras.

7. Cooked whole grain cereals—millet, quinoa, or buckwheat with nut butter drizzled on top

8. Cook scrambled eggs and then stir cooked quinoa into eggs to warm. Season with Herbamare seasoning salt.

9. Dinner leftovers

Phase 1 Snacks:

1. Small handful of raw nuts or seeds—almonds, pecans, filberts, pumpkin seeds, sunflower seeds
2. Celery, pepper, or carrot sticks and other veggies plain or can be dipped in tahini (ground sesame seeds), almond butter, or other nut butter.
3. Homemade plain yogurt (fermented 24 hours) with stevia sweetener. If store-bought plain yogurt, stir in one or two capsules of probiotics (good bacteria). Only eat yogurt if tolerated—if unsure avoid until symptoms subside then test
4. Avocado + fresh tomatoes + apple cider vinegar (or fresh lemon/ lime juice) + olive oil
5. Warm artichoke hearts (plain not marinated), black olives with a splash of lemon and chopped dill
6. Leftovers from the previous meal
7. Cup of broth (chicken or veggie) with added veggies and herbs
8. A salad—throw nuts on top. Salad dressing—apple cider vinegar, fresh lemon juice or fresh lime juice with olive oil, flax seed oil or grape seed oil (oils should be cold pressed or virgin)

*Always listen to your body. If you eat something and it gives you stomach discomfort, eliminate it from your diet and test it again later. If it continues to bother you, avoid it.

Main Meal Ideas

To avoid boredom, plan ahead and cook with a variety of vegetables, meats (or other vegetarian proteins), herbs, spices, and flavors. The following list will give you a few ideas. You can find specific recipes online, in books at your local library, or in the books that I have recommended:

Curry Meat or Veggie Dishes	• Thai green or red curry paste—(no peanuts), virgin coconut oil—not coconut milk • Curry, cumin, coriander, turmeric, etc. • Many of these spices have antifungal and anti-inflammatory properties. Avoid soya sauce during the Initial Phase.
Stir Fries	• Use a variety of vegetables—onions, bok choy, Chinese cabbage, peppers, celery, sesame oil, fresh garlic and ginger, salt and pepper or Herbamare • Add cooked meat or meat substitute • Serve over brown rice, quinoa, buckwheat or spaghetti squash
Greek	• Dill, garlic, cumin • Chicken, lamb, or pork souvlaki • Greek salad minus the feta cheese Use lemon juice, or apple cider vinegar, with olive oil, oregano and pepper. Plain olives are okay.

Mexican Taco Salad	• Veggies—chopped fresh peppers, onions, tomatoes, homemade guacamole (cilantro, fresh lime juice, Herbamare, fresh garlic, avocado) • Extra lean ground beef or other ground meat (cooked tofu or beans if vegetarian) seasoned with cumin, garlic, paprika, chilli powder, salt, etc. (grass fed and organic meat is best—see the meat section in the above chart) • Brown rice or quinoa • Homemade salsa—fresh tomatoes, onions, herbs, apple cider vinegar, or fresh lemon juice to make it tart *If beans give you lots of gas, avoid them during the Initial Phase. You want to minimize fermentation while killing the enemy. Digestive enzymes can also minimize fermentation.*
Italian Tomato Sauce	• Organic tomatoes, fresh or dried oregano, basil, thyme, rosemary, and garlic • Can add cooked lean meat (grass fed, organic is best) beans or cooked tofu if vegetarian. • This sauce can be put on cooked spaghetti squash, brown rice, quinoa, or buckwheat.
Homemade soups	French onion (no cheese or bread), vegetable borscht (substitute yogurt for the cream or just omit it and replace apple cider vinegar for the white vinegar), chicken vegetable (add rice, quinoa or buckwheat)

Homemade stews	Include all non-starchy veggies and meat or protein substitute. Just omit the white potatoes.
Salads	• Vary the veggies, nuts (oven roasted nuts on a salad are delicious), olives, avocado, meats or meat substitutes, salad dressings. • Cold-cooked quinoa works well in salads. • Herb salad dressing—Use fresh lemon or lime juice, or apple cider vinegar, olive oil (or other oils listed on page 128) and fresh or dried herbs such as dill, basil, parsley, mint, garlic, cayenne, etc. • Tahini salad dressing—Mix tahini, water, lemon or lime juice, or apple cider vinegar, olive oil, and a dash of seasoning salt, such as Herbamare, to the desired consistency and taste. This makes a very tasty dressing. • Cucumber dressing—Blend cucumber, oil, dill, garlic, and cayenne in a blender. Eat within one hour. Do not store.

Tips:
- Avoid eating foods that cause a lot of fermentation (gas). With gas comes the production of chemicals, some of which have a negative effect on our immune system. During the Initial Phase, you are killing the enemy and want to support your immune system to help you with this process.
- When you include a protein and a carb for breakfast (ex: millet with almond butter drizzled on top) you will be satisfied for several hours. If you just eat the whole grain cereal without protein you may be hungry much sooner.
- Make sure to plan ahead and include a variety of homemade

soups, stir fries, salads and other dishes to avoid boredom.

- Enjoy winter squashes in place of starchy carbs like potatoes.
- At least half of your meal should be made up of a variety of non-starchy veggies.
- During the Initial Phase avoid anything that is really sweet. Some programs allow sweet potato during the Initial Phase. I found that it set me back during that part of the program. Listen to your body. You are better off being stricter with the program, getting results faster and then testing foods once your health has improved dramatically.
- Avoid using a lot of stevia. It is much healthier if you become accustomed to foods that aren't overly sweet. As you wean yourself from sweets, your cravings will subside and then you won't have to struggle with this in the future.
- Remain on this part of the program as long as necessary. This part of the program can also be followed if you have had fungal overgrowth in the past, are under lots of stress and want to avoid a relapse of yeast overgrowth. This eating plan includes foods that are nutritious and do not encourage fungal growth.

RECOVERY PHASE: DURATION: 2 WEEKS–6 MONTHS

As the yeast overgrowth has been treated and symptoms of fungal overgrowth are no longer apparent, the Recovery Phase can be followed. This phase includes a healthy but less restrictive eating plan and promotes optimal functioning and health in the various systems in the body. Ultimately, it's a whole food eating plan that is full of nutrition, easy to digest, and does not encourage fungal growth. During the Recovery Phase, continue to take high-quality plant derived nutritional supplements, a potent probiotic (good bacteria), and maintain a healthy lifestyle (see Pillar #4 on page 181). This approach will support optimal digestive health, immune function, endocrine function and optimal function of all other systems in the body, which in turn will discourage the invasion of yeast in the future.

This part of the program allows you to be a little less strict with your eating plan but still promotes strengthening of your immune system.

Recovery Phase Tips:
Eat the same foods found in Initial Phase, but now add the following foods *occasionally* (keep total servings of processed carbs to a minimum). Remember to pay attention to how you feel: your energy level and the state of your digestive system. If symptoms begin to return, then go back to the Initial Phase of the program and stick to it for a longer period of time.

Enjoy the following occasionally:
- Apple—less sweet variety
- Papayas
- Rice cakes with nut butter—no more than a couple per day
- Whole grain corn tortillas if tolerated
- Corn chips if tolerated—a treat on a weekend
- Whole grain gluten free pancakes, muffins, waffles (brown rice, quinoa, buckwheat, etc.)
- Small amounts of goat cheese if tolerated
- * Use caution with corn. Many people do not tolerate it. If you re-introduce corn and tolerate it, eat one or two servings per week.

RECIPES
Brown Rice Muffins—Basic Recipe
Mix together:
4 cups brown rice flour
¾ cup rice bran or wheat bran if tolerated
2 tsp. baking powder (no aluminium)
2 tsp. baking soda
1 heaping tsp. cinnamon (optional)

In a separate bowl beat well together:

3 eggs, beaten

4-5 smashed bananas—not over-ripe

1 tbsp. natural vanilla extract

½ cup of vegetable oil

Approximately 2 cups of water, unsweetened rice milk or almond milk if tolerated

Add the dry ingredients alternately with the two cups of liquid into the liquid mixture. Stir in a few blueberries or chopped nuts if you choose (optional). Batter should be the consistency of thick pancake batter, so add a bit more water or liquid as needed. Place the batter in paper muffin cups in a muffin baking pan or directly into a greased muffin pan. Bake at 350° oven for 25–30 min.

These muffins are best if you eat them fresh and freeze the extras. Thaw and warm in a toaster oven. This is a great basic recipe that you can modify (for example—add flax seed, berries or nuts, etc.). During the Surveillance Phase you can add a handful or two of organic raisins, currents, or unsweetened cranberries.

Brown Rice Pancakes

Mix together:

2 cups of brown rice flour

¾ cup of rice bran or wheat bran if tolerated

2 tsp. of baking powder (no aluminium)

1 tsp. of baking soda

1 tsp. cinnamon (optional)

In a separate bowl mix:

3 beaten eggs

1 tbsp. vanilla

Melted butter—about ⅛ – ¼ cup of real butter in a frying pan on low heat—don't brown the butter.

1-2 cups of fresh or partially thawed berries (optional)

Add the egg mixture and about two cups of water (or unsweetened almond or rice milk) to the dry mixture. Stir well. Stir in melted butter. The batter should not be too thick or too runny. Adjust the consistency to what you like. If the batter is too runny you can always add a bit more rice flour to thicken. Fold in berries. Cook pancakes in frying pan and turn when bubbles form, pop open and stay open, and when the bottom is brown.

These are delicious and freeze really well to preserve. They make a quick breakfast—try spreading nut butter on pancakes and you will be satisfied for hours. Don't binge on these, just eat enough that you are satisfied. Binging on carbs will encourage a return of yeast overgrowth.

To-Die-For Belgian Rice Waffles
Yes, I realize that there is a little butter in this recipe, but our family loves it and reserves it for special occasions!

4 eggs
½ tsp. salt
½ cup real butter melted
1 tbsp. sugar
2 cups brown rice flour
1 cup unsweetened almond milk, rice milk or water
1 tbsp. baking powder (no aluminium)
1 tsp. natural vanilla extract

Beat the eggs and sugar together until light and foamy. Add cooled melted butter, milk (or water), vanilla and mix together. Sift rice flour and baking powder together (we just stir them together with a whisk). Add blended dry ingredients to egg mixture. Add salt and beat well. Bake in a Belgian waffle maker. Makes about 10 waffles.

Serve waffles with real whipped cream (can use stevia or a minimal amount of sugar) and unsweetened fresh or thawed berries. Absolutely delicious!!

Once the yeast issue is under control, you can add a drizzle of natural maple syrup over the whipped cream and berries …mmmm!

Do the following if you are in the Recovery Phase and want to minimize the effect of your indulgence. In a small jar (approximately 2 cups) add one cup water, one tsp. of psyllium husks and open one or two capsules of digestive enzymes. Place the lid on the jar, shake the mixture and drink just before eating the waffles.

SURVEILLANCE PHASE: DURATION—INDEFINITELY

Congratulations! You have reached this phase of the program when your energy has returned, the fungal symptoms have subsided for an adequate amount of time and your immune system is strong. Your health care professional has confirmed that the yeast is now back to minimal levels in your body.

If you have suffered with Candida overgrowth for years and have recently completed the anti-Candida program, it is important to realize that you are still susceptible to flare-ups of yeast growth in the future. I have been coaching clients and researching this topic for more than twenty years and have not found a complete cure for this condition. This is because, as discussed earlier, yeast has the ability to establish an extensive root system deep in our tissues and has the ability to form biofilms; both make it difficult to get all the yeast out of the tissues. Also, re-establishing the healthy terrain in the gut takes time and effort.

You choose the quality of life that you want. If you want to live a vibrant life, do not go back to your old nutritional habits and lifestyle or the yeast overgrowth will likely flourish again.

Tips for the Surveillance Phase:

- Continue to eat a variety of whole foods, where at least 50% of your plate consists of non-starchy vegetables—include raw veggies with each meal.
- Eat three meals each day with healthy snacks in between. The types of foods eaten in this phase will be similar to the Initial and Recovery phase of the Candida program but you can have an

occasional moderate cheat. When you eat whole foods you will find that you will feel satisfied. You will be able to eat whenever you are hungry, but without the fear of weight gain.

- With each meal, eat just enough complex carbs to maintain health and weight, but not enough to encourage yeast growth. Remember that even complex carbs can cause blood sugar levels to rise too high if the serving size is too large. This will promote fungal growth.
- Avoid eating processed carbs (anything made from ground grain or flour) during the week. If you must have a modest indulgence on the weekend, keep it to just that. The less processed carbs you eat, the less you will crave them. Pay attention to how you are feeling. If old symptoms return, cut back in this area.
- Monitor your lifestyle. Make sure that you offset stress with adequate water, nutrition, sleep and exercise. Make sure that you have down time and don't forget a healthy dose of sunshine.
- Continue to supplement with a potent probiotic and plant-sourced nutritional supplements (see page 77).

Candida Program for Children

When working with children it is important to do your homework and work with an experienced health care professional. Do not take the advice of a stranger on the Internet. I recommend that you follow the advice of a medical doctor or naturopath that has experience in this area. The following information that I am sharing comes from my own personal experience and subsequent success in dealing with fungal overgrowth in my children. I have read many books by different doctors and have worked with health care professionals when dealing with my children's health.

I am a wellness coach, not a health care professional and this information is not intended to advise treatment of your child. I am simply sharing this information with you for educational purposes so that you will have some background, understanding and insight; and be better equipped to work with an experienced health care professional. *The Complete Candida Yeast Guidebook* by Jeanne Marie Martin with Dr. Zolton Rona has a section for dietary suggestions for children. Dr. Fred Pescatore also has an excellent book called *Feed Your Kids Well*. Both can be ordered through your local health food store or online through Amazon.

Modifying your child's food preferences can be a challenge. Children's taste buds are more sensitive to flavors and they don't really understand the idea of treating yeast overgrowth. A few parents have told me that they just can't get their young child to eat healthy foods. I then ask them a simple question: if your child's life depended on it could you find a way? Of course the answer is yes. And for the record—yes, the quality and length of your child's life is significantly impacted by their nutritional habits. Here are some of the tricks that I have used to encourage my kids to eat healthy foods when they were young.

Six easy tips to get your kids to eat and learn to like their veggies:

1. It will definitely be easiest for you and your child if you begin teaching them to appreciate a variety of flavors when they are old enough to start eating solid foods. When your child is ready for solids, introduce a variety of vegetables and other foods (one at a time and at the appropriate age). I found it convenient to steam several cups of one organic vegetable, cool it, purée it (in its cooking water) and freeze in stainless steel ice cube trays. When frozen, put the veggie cubes in a container in the freezer (preferably not plastic). You can also do this with meats and fruits. This makes it quick and easy to give your child a healthy variety of foods that aren't overly processed.

2. If your child doesn't like the taste of certain veggies at the start, put some of the veggie or other food on a spoon and dip the end of the spoon in a home-made unsweetened fruit purée like apple sauce. The idea here is to dip the end of the spoon, not cover it. You want the child to still be able to taste the veggie and eventually become

accustomed to the flavours. Over time, slowly decrease the amount of fruit purée on the end of the spoon until they are eating the vegetable on its own.

3. If your child is a toddler or preschooler and you have allowed them to develop poor eating habits, you may experience a bit more resistance, but you owe it to them to persevere. If your child doesn't want to eat the food that you have prepared and you have encouraged them for some time, just set the food aside. When they come back hungry a short while later, don't give them the processed snack that they want, offer them the food that they refused. If they are hungry enough, chances are they will eat it eventually.

4. Another trick that works well is to offer a reward. If your child is old enough to understand this, let them know that as soon as they have finished eating, you will play their favourite game with them. Get them thinking about the game and it is amazing how their mind is so focused on the reward that they will eat the food with little or no hassle. You know your child and what motivates him or her. Use your imagination.

5. Make sure to give your children positive reinforcement when they eat foods they don't like, and when they are old enough, explain that the veggies and other whole foods will make them run faster, play harder... again, whatever is important to your child.

6. If your child struggles with a certain food, work a deal with them. Tell them that they only have to eat so many bites. This way you are still giving them the opportunity to get used to new foods (especially certain veggies) and they feel that they are getting a break. You won't want to play this game all the time, just in certain instances where you can see that they are really struggling with the particular food. If you persist, they will get used to most vegetables and whole foods and will even learn to appreciate them.

Important note

- Do not send your child to school with money to buy lunch. Instead, prepare lunch at home. When they are old enough, get them involved in preparing their own lunch the night before. You'll be taking more control over the quality of food they eat as well as teaching them an important life skill. I realize that everyone is busy, but the lunch provided at school will not support your child's optimal health. I have been a teacher for more than 10 years and I see what kids are eating. Schools are making an effort to provide healthier choices for students, but for the most part many of the healthier choices are still not nutritious enough.

A child that is used to eating a variety of vegetables and whole foods will be much healthier and chances are they will not be a fussy or picky eater.

INITIAL PHASE GUIDELINES FOR CHILDREN

- Choose whole raw fruit that is not too sweet. Best choices are apples, berries, kiwis, avocados, papayas, white grapefruits, and Japanese pear apples. Choose fruit that is organic where available and avoid non-organic fruit from the Dirty Dozen list. Fruit should not be over-ripe. Avoid all fruit juice, canned fruit or fruit snacks and other processed fruits.
- Best choice for whole grains—gluten free grains such as brown rice, millet, quinoa, amaranth and buckwheat. (See recipe for brown rice pancakes, muffins, etc.)
- Avoid all dairy products (except real butter). Homemade yogurt is okay if tolerated but it must be fermented for at least 24 hours.
- Enjoy unsweetened rice, or almond milk (if no allergies). Avoid soya milk as it has been shown to impair the absorption of minerals. Remember to supplement with a good calcium supplement if you are avoiding dairy products.
- All the vegetables, meats, nuts and good fats listed in the Initial Phase for adults will work for children also as long as they are old enough to eat it and do not have allergies to it.
- Good fats are important. Use real butter and virgin olive oil, grape flax and coconut oil—cold pressed not hydrogenated.

- What to drink? Get your child accustomed to drinking filtered water. This should be the most important beverage of the day.

*The main difference between an adult and a child's version of the Initial Phase of the Candida program is that complex carbs from specific fruits and grains are not restricted for children during the program. Children require the energy and calories from the specific carbohydrates because their bodies are actively growing.

Tips:
- School-aged children can pack home-made soups, stews or other meals in a thermos.
- Make a sandwich for your child from home-made rice pancakes (see the recipe section).
- Many children with Candida overgrowth develop food sensitivities or allergies and these foods must be avoided. Some of these reactions can be severe. As the fungal overgrowth is dealt with, many of the sensitivities and allergies tend to settle down. Anaphylaxic reactions usually persist and foods that cause these reactions should never be tested without the guidance of a medical professional.

2. KILL THE ENEMY

Killing the enemy is accomplished simultaneously with the Initial Phase of the Candida program. This involves using various therapeutic agents that kill the yeast.

At this time there is no permanent cure for yeast/fungal overgrowth. Yes, I've said it again, and if someone tries to tell you differently they are misinformed or just telling you this in hopes of selling you something. There is no quick fix or simple pill that will cure you so that you can go back to your old ways. If you truly understand this you will save yourself time, money and plenty of frustration. With that said, it is possible to knock back the population of yeast/fungi and other parasites in your body to the point where they no longer cause disease symptoms and you can enjoy an excellent quality of life. Once balance is restored, you will be able to have an occasional cheat and it won't set you back. If your desire is to keep your new-found freedom in wellness for many years to come, then you should never return to your old ways again. You choose the level of wellness you want.

You choose what is more important to you: satisfying your taste buds from junk food cravings, feeling lousy and shortening your lifespan, or living an active vibrant life and adding many high quality years to your longevity. If your choice is to live an active vibrant life, I am confident that over time you will gain a new appreciation for fresh, whole natural foods and won't want to go back to processed lifeless food-like substances. Just give your taste buds time to adjust.

Killing the enemy means war: the war of reclaiming your body and your health. Long lasting success cannot be accomplished by taking a single pill. The key to your success will be your dedication in the Initial Phase of the diet, taking a therapeutic agent (or therapeutic agents) to reduce the population of bad guys, and building up your immune system through nutrition and lifestyle. If you omit one part of this formula you will have limited results.

It is important to deal with dysbiosis as soon as possible. The sooner it is dealt with the easier it is to treat. Treating dysbiosis can be accomplished in one of two ways:

1. By using a more natural, gentle approach
2. By using a more aggressive approach

The gentle natural approach to killing

This approach is for those suffering with mild or moderate dysbiosis; individuals not plagued with disease. They may have recently finished a prescription of antibiotics or used antibiotics in the past. Their complaints are often related to one or more of the following symptoms (from the list on page 112): digestive issues (constipation, gas, diarrhea, stomach aches, or acid reflux), allergies, chronic sinus issues, vaginitis in women, jock itch in men, nail fungus, chronic sinusitis, and/or dandruff. People in this group are in the early stages of fungal overgrowth. They are aware that something is not right as their body gives them minor warning signs. They just haven't stepped into chronic disease yet and won't have to if they deal with this now!

Protocol for mild-moderate dysbiosis

1. Follow the Initial Phase of the diet for at least the minimum recommended length of time—longer if necessary.
2. Rotate herbal antifungals and eat foods that have antifungal properties or use therapeutic probiotics (probiotics that kill yeast).
3. Supplement with plant-based enzyme supplements. Enzymes aid in the digestion of food.
4. Take a potent probiotic supplement—if you decide to use a therapeutic probiotic (see page 150) then skip this for the short term.
5. Supplement with natural plant-based nutrients—including glyconutrients.
6. Manage stress through a healthy lifestyle. (see Pillar #4 page 181)
7. Get adequate sleep. (see Pillar #4 page 181)
8. Women—avoid the birth control pill. (see Section Three—Women's Health Issues page 194)
9. Teenagers—avoid antibiotics for acne.

The more aggressive approach

If you believe that dysbiosis has been a chronic condition in your life for years, the type and length of treatment may be more involved as the yeast has likely moved to other parts of the body, established an extensive root system deep in the tissues and built biofilms which resist treatment.

Individuals in this group usually have symptoms that range from the mild to moderate group and could also suffer with chronic disease, pain, debilitating fatigue, a suppressed immune system, difficulty with focus and other aspects of cognition, depression, and/or hormonal imbalances just to name a few.

If this is the case, you may want to follow a more aggressive protocol. The same protocol for mild to moderate dysbiosis applies, but the Initial Phase of the diet must be followed as long as necessary. The Initial Phase outlines a healthy eating plan which can be maintained indefinitely. You are the only one who can gauge how long you should remain on it. If you follow the diet for the minimum recommended time and when you start to re-introduce foods you notice that old symptoms slowly begin to return, then you should remain on the Initial Phase diet for a longer period of time. Listen to your body. It will let you know when it has had enough time to heal.

You will want to work aggressively with natural antifungals or discuss the option of using a pharmaceutical antifungal with your doctor. Pharmaceutical antifungals can be effective if used for a short term (a few months) and if your doctor is able to match the correct drug with the correct strain of yeast/fungus. Remember, yeast/fungi are very adaptive and tend to become resistant to drugs relatively quickly, so the drug approach is useful to get you out of the crisis but is not an effective long term solution. Also, pharmaceuticals have side effects and many antifungal drugs require that your doctor monitor your liver function while taking the drug.

Anti-fungal foods

Nature provides many foods that discourage yeast/fungal growth in the body.

Antifungal Foods and Spices	
• Raw garlic	• Apple cider vinegar
• Virgin coconut oil	• Olive oil
• Non-starchy vegetables which are rich in phytochemicals and antioxidants	• Raw carrots
	• Spices: curries, coriander, turmeric, cinnamon, cloves

Herb or Agent	Mode of Action
Garlic	• Antibacterial, antifungal, antiviral, antiparasitic and anticancer activities • Prebiotic (food for probiotics)
Olive Leaf	• Antibacterial, antiviral, antifungal, antiparasitic
Oil of Oregano	• Antibacterial, antiviral, antifungal, antiparasitic
Acemannan found in Aloe vera	• Antibacterial, antiviral, antifungal, anticancer
Golden Seal	• Antibacterial, antifungal, antiviral, antiparasitic and anticancer activities • Laxative
Pau d'Arco bark (tea)	• Antibacterial, antifungal, antiviral, antiparasitic and anticancer activities, blood thinner
Caprilic acid	• Antibacterial, antifungal
Grapefruit seed extract	• Antibacterial, antifungal, antiviral
Chlorophyll	• Anticancer, antioxidant, antimutagenic (mutagenic agents can cause a mutation in DNA), reduce the bioavailability and/or activity of ingested aflatoxin (mycotoxin)
Enzymes	• Specific enzymes that poke holes in the cell wall of the yeast and digest the protein in yeast (cellulase, hemicellulase, and protease)

*Note: If you take any medication, consult with your doctor before taking an herb or other therapeutic agent. Some herbs interact with certain medications. As mentioned, pharmacists can also be very helpful.

It is important to work with an experienced health care professional when using antifungal herbs and agents. The health care professional will ensure that you take enough of the therapeutic agent so the treatment will be effective. Also, antifungals should be rotated every few days to ensure that the yeast/fungi or other microbe does not become resistant to the treatment. Although medicinal herbs come from nature, they still act like natural medicines in the body and some will react negatively with pharmaceutical medications. Medicinal herbs should not be taken indefinitely as their effectiveness may diminish and some herbs have toxic effects on the body if taken for a long period of time.

Acemannan found that Aloe vera is an exception and can be taken indefinitely. It provides a nutrient—a glyconutrient (discussed in the nutrition section of the book)—which supports cell-to-cell communication, optimal brain function and immune function.

The goal in using natural antifungals is to use them just long enough to reduce the numbers of yeast/fungi in the body and then to repopulate the GI tract with the good guys (probiotics). This must be done in conjunction with supporting optimal immune function because we want our immune system to fight the infection also. For best results follow all the steps in the Protocol for Mild to Moderate Yeast Overgrowth (page 145).

Using therapeutic probiotics to kill the enemy
Although antifungal herbs and drugs can be effective, many people complain of relapses over time. This program does knock back the population of yeast but may not restore a complete balance.

I believe that our best hope for controlling dysbiosis will come from the world of probiotics. There has been a growing interest in this field of study in recent years and several effective therapeutic products have been introduced to the market. There are basically two types of probiotics.

The Muscle Heads
The most common probiotic supplement contains several standard strains of bacteria that normally live in our GI tract. These are the good guys and include many of the Lactobacillus strains of bacteria

such as acidophilus and bifidus. I like to think of the good guys as the muscle heads; the guys at the gym that are all pumped up.

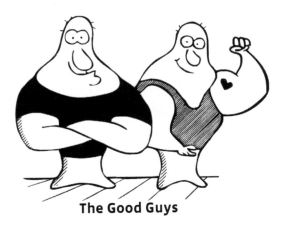

The Good Guys

These buffed good guys reach the yeast and other parasites in the GI tract and fight with them for space and nutrients. This might look like a typical brawl where the good guys attempt to crowd out the bad guys. If you take a probiotic that isn't potent enough, you may not notice any improvement because the bad guys outnumber the good guys. This would be an unfair fight: too many bad and not enough good.

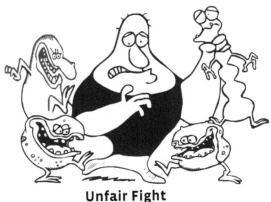

Unfair Fight

In the past, I have used many probiotics and didn't really notice a difference in the health of my GI tract. This may have been either because I wasn't taking a strong enough dose or that the units of active bacteria in the supplement were less than what was listed on the label. Just because a supplement says that each capsule contains 9 billion active organisms, you really have no way of knowing that this is true unless the product has been tested by a third party (independent lab).

I have coached clients who have used probiotic supplements that may contain on average 10 billion living organisms per capsule and even though they increased the dose, the benefits were minimal. I have also worked with clients who tried newer probiotic supplements containing several hundred billion living organisms per serving and finally notice improvements to the health of their GI tract. It is so important to take the appropriate dose and the correct strains of pro-biotics to ensure success. An experienced health care professional can be invaluable.

Again, children are resilient and most recover from dysbiosis quickly by using a whole food eating plan, avoiding dairy, gluten and sugar, taking nutritional supplements and supplementing with an effective probiotic.

The Military

These probiotics possess therapeutic properties as they contain strains of bacteria that are also considered good guys, but they are more like soldiers in the military. Many of these strains are not found in large amounts in the human GI tract. They are predators of yeast/fungi, bad bacteria and other bad bugs. Their sole mission is to seek out and destroy the enemy as they pass through the GI tract. As they approach yeast/fungi and other harmful microbes they kill the bad guys. They open fire on the bad guys not just bruising them but actually killing them. Yeast/fungi and other bad microbes do not become resistant as easily to this type of therapy as it uses a predator/prey model found in nature.

As this is a relatively new and growing field, it is important to work with an experienced health care professional who will recommend

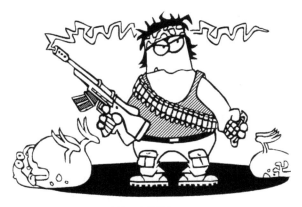

The Military

the most effective blend of probiotics. The future of probiotics is very exciting and bright. My hope is that as dysbiosis and silent infections become more accepted and understood, better tests will be available to help us determine which microbe or microbes are making us sick, and the treatment will include a specific blend of probiotics to target the bad bugs that are responsible for our illness.

Caution: it may not be feasible to take antifungal herbs that also kill bacteria (such as the ones listed on page 147) while you are taking therapeutic probiotics. These herbs will kill bad bacteria but will also damage the therapeutic probiotics. If you choose take an antifungal herb treatment, do this before you start the probiotics and then discontinue it while you are on the therapeutic probiotics.

3. RE-ESTABLISH THE GOOD GUYS

This part of the program takes time. It would be great if we could just swallow a pill for 5–10 days and restore the trillions of good or friendly bacteria that were destroyed when we swallowed the antibiotic for 5–10 days. Each time you swallow a probiotic some of the good guys do make it to the GI tract but many are destroyed by the strong acid and digestive juices found in the stomach and digestive system, and thus don't survive the journey to the GI tract.

Some probiotic supplements are *enteric coated* which means that they are better able to withstand the strong acid in the stomach. Probiotic supplements often include food or prebiotics for the good guys so they don't starve while being stored. Fructo-oligosaccharides, (FOS) and arabino-oligosaccharides (AOS) are two examples of food sources that may be listed on the label.

4. SURVEILLANCE

At this time you have finished the intensive part of the program and you are feeling great! This is reward time! You should celebrate and treat yourself. Pick a treat that is health-promoting like some new clothes, a massage, a trip or holiday—even if just for a weekend.

Your energy is high, your digestive system is happy, and many of your complaints have subsided or vanished. Others have asked what you are doing differently because they have noticed a change in you. They comment on how great you look! Many clients have told me that they had felt lousy for so long that they had forgotten how great they could feel.

The surveillance part of the program continues for the rest of your life. It is now your job to guard your health. You are aware when stress is high in your life. In these situations you must make adjustments in your lifestyle to protect your health so that you never have to return to the place where you started.

High stress, pregnancy, antibiotic use, lack of exercise, eating processed foods (especially carbs), prolonged lack of sleep and other factors will promote the re-occurrence of fungal overgrowth in our body. Now you are aware of how great you feel when you are healthy and you remember how lousy you felt when you were plagued with fungal growth. My hope is that the avoidance of that pain will motivate you to follow the habits of a Wellness Champion. It did for me.

It's all about give and take. In times of high stress you may want to follow the Initial Phase of the program and get more sleep. This doesn't mean that you can never have a glass of wine again or a dessert on a special occasion. It does mean that you give yourself occasional modest indulgences that do not jeopardize your wellness. Your level of wellness is affected by many things and is constantly changing. It is a continuum; you choose the level of wellness that you want.

Tips to control yeast:

- Do not go sleep deprived for long periods of time. Adequate sleep is vital for a healthy immune system. If you don't get eight hours of sleep, get caught up the following night.
- Manage stress. During times of increased stress move back to the Initial Phase of the program and focus on the Four Pillars of Wellness more seriously.
- Do a Candida cleanse (Initial Phase) once or twice a year as needed. Follow the program strictly.
- Listen to your body. If you recognize symptoms returning, go back to the Recovery or Initial Phase of the program.
- Avoid binging on carbs or alcohol. North Americans eat too many servings of grains each day, especially processed carbs. Eat just enough whole grain carbs to maintain a healthy weight but not enough to encourage fungal growth.
- Exercise is very important, especially aerobic exercise.
- Get some sun exposure each day if possible. Avoid long periods of sun exposure especially when UV levels are high. Sunshine is very important in maintaining a strong immune system.
- Establish a nutritional supplement program that is high quality and plant-sourced. If you optimize nutrition, your immune system—and your body in general—will work at its peak. Glyconutrients are important in optimal immune function.
- Many people have reported benefits from using an infrared sauna. This may be due to the increased body temperature (similar to having a fever) which discourages bacterial, viral and yeast growth, and causes sweating and the release of toxins from the body.

- You may re-introduce gluten and dairy products into your eating plan again, but with caution. You may find that you do better if you only eat gluten once or twice a week or avoid it all together, likewise with dairy. You may want to continue to avoid dairy, other than plain yogurt (with an acidophilus capsule) and small amounts of goat cheese.

Protect the health of your GI tract

The old saying, "disease begins in the gut" holds a lot of truth. The vast majority of us will deal with some type of digestive issue in our lifetime. Here we will summarize how to maintain the health and integrity of your GI tract. Most of us have ignored this area for years but a healthful GI tract is critical for optimal health.

Follow these simple steps to optimize the health of your GI tract:

1. Don't ignore the symptoms of dysbiosis. If you are experiencing gas, bloating, pain, constipation or diarrhea, do not ignore these symptoms; they are often your first warning signs. If you chose to ignore them, these symptoms will worsen over time and other aspects of your health will be affected. If your symptoms are serious, visit a health care provider to obtain a proper diagnosis and then begin working at improving the health of your GI tract.
2. Eliminate daily. It is really important that you have at least one bowel movement each day. Eliminating waste is just as important as taking nutrients in. If you are not eliminating at least once a day, waste will build up and place undue stress on your liver and other organs. Normal stool should be brown to light brown, cylinder shaped and formed but not hard or too soft.

Five simple steps to promote regular elimination:

1. Drink adequate filtered water throughout the day. A trick that works well is to drink a large glass of warm water upon arising first thing in the morning, before you do anything else. This stimulates

the GI tract to eliminate.

2. Physical exercise such as walking, running, biking, etc. helps to promote elimination.

3. If you have issues with constipation, avoid all dairy, gluten grains, and processed carbs. Eat smaller whole food meals more often. Incorporate lots of non-starchy veggies. If your GI tract is inflamed, you may want to choose vegetables that don't aggravate the inflammation. Also try lightly steaming the vegetables. The inflammation will subside as the infection is dealt with and the gut heals.

4. Get adequate sleep. Sleep deprivation affects the immune system and the digestive system in a big way. If you are trying to heal the gut, adequate sleep is vital. The hours of sleep before midnight are the most rejuvenating. If you are dealing with health issues and feel that you need more sleep, listen to your body. A quick nap in the afternoon is great for your health.

5. Use fiber with adequate amounts of water to promote elimination. Prescription laxatives can be habit forming, meaning they make your GI tract lazy so that, over time, you become more constipated. Look for fiber blends that contain psyllium, acacia fiber, fennel seed, slippery elm, marshmallow, etc. If you use a fiber blend, make sure you drink enough water with the fiber or it could make you more constipated. Also, don't take fiber with medication or supplements because fiber will bind to them making them unavailable to your body.

Once your health has returned, you will experience a new-found freedom. Now you must eat to live; not live to eat. Your food should be the fuel that allows you to live life to the fullest. Now go out, live and pay it forward!

I am not getting results

There are several reasons why you may not be getting the results you desire from the program. I have included them, starting with the most common:

- Cheating on the eating plan—knowingly or unknowingly? The yeast overgrowth will feed on normal blood sugar levels, and will really prosper if you eat the wrong carbs or even too much of the right carbs. It is vital to follow the eating program until you have the desired outcome. A few little cheats will stop you from reaching your goal.

- How are your stress levels? Are you overworked? Do you have enough down time? Is your life in balance? Are you getting enough sleep? High levels of emotional, physiological and/or physical stress together with a lack of sleep will hinder your body's ability to heal. Getting at least eight hours of sleep is essential for your body to heal and restore itself.

- You may have other parasites that are suppressing your immune system and preventing you from recovering. Some examples include worms, flukes, mycoplasmas, plasmodium, mycobacterium, protozoa, amoeba and many other harmful organisms. Work with a qualified health care professional to determine if should do a parasite cleanse. The success of a parasite cleanse depends on taking the right medication or blend of herbs for the specific parasite and also taking the correct dosage and for a sufficient amount of time. If a person has lived with chronic yeast overgrowth for years, other parasites often establish themselves in the GI tract: yeast overgrowth suppresses the immune system making the body more vulnerable to other parasites. Bad microbes will also live in yeast biofilms where they can hide from our immune system, treatments, and other good bacteria that would otherwise destroy them.

- Yeast overgrowth that resists treatment can also be the result of heavy metal toxicity—especially from mercury (see the mercury section in the chapter about toxins). Work with an experienced health care provider if you feel that you may have heavy metal toxicity.

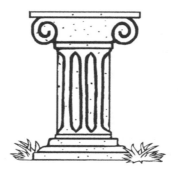

Pillar #3
Minimize Your Toxin Load

TOXINS, TOXINS EVERYWHERE!

There is no denying that the over 80,000 synthetic chemicals[169] introduced over the past 50 years have impacted our lives radically. Synthetic chemicals have revolutionized everything from the interior of our vehicles to providing us with near perfect produce. Most of us have not paid much attention to the fact that these chemicals might harm us. We tend to rationalize: "sure, they may carry a strong odor, but surely our government wouldn't allow companies to include chemicals in their products unless there were safe... right?" Unfortunately most chemicals are presumed safe until proven harmful.[170] Less than 10% of the 80,000 synthetic chemicals on record have been tested for safety in adults and less than 5% have been tested for safety in children.[171] Not only is the sheer number of untested chemicals a concern but their interaction can enhance adverse health effects.[172]

But we can't place all the blame on the government. Over the past 10 years there has been a growing awareness of the increasing toxic load in our environment, yet we are resistant to change because the chemicals in question make our lives easier and provide us with luxuries that we believe are hard to give up.

One can find thousands of scientific papers online and accordingly, it would take much more than one book to give this topic justice. My goal is to share a sampling of current research in a few key areas that impact your life, in hopes that the facts will shock you into action. I have been very health conscious for the past 20 plus years, yet the research that I am about to share with you has motivated me to work harder in this area. I encourage you to research further on your own. The impact of environmental chemicals on our health and the health of our children is so serious that we must take action now!

About 3000 chemicals are produced at quantities of more than one million pounds per year, yet little information is available as to their potential harmful effects on human learning and development. There is a strong indication that 200 of these chemicals are neurotoxins and approximately 1000 are suspected to negatively affect the human nervous system. The neurotoxic effect of more than 75,000 chemicals is not known at this time.[173]

Hundreds of these chemicals are building up in our tissues and no expert fully understands the consequences to our health. Several studies have tested individuals from across North America and found more than 200 substances showing up in their blood and urine. The participants in the studies were average people. None of them worked with chemicals on the job or in chemical factories.[174]

The Centers for Disease Control and Prevention[175] echoed this same message in their report, *National Report on Human Exposure to Environmental Chemicals*. They found that most participants in the study had detectable levels of commonly used industrial chemical groups such as:

- Polybrominated diphenyl ethers (PBDEs) or fire retardants,
- Bisphenol A (BPA) found in many plastics such as toys, beverage containers, dental sealants, lining in tin cans
- Perfluorinated chemicals (PFCs) found in nonstick pans in their blood and urine

This report also found widespread exposure to heavy metal mercury as well as acrylamide—a chemical formed from cooking carbohydrates at a high temperature, or consumed by smoking cigarettes.

TOXINS & OUR CHILDREN

As parents, our deepest desire is to provide an environment that allows our children to develop to their full potential in all aspects of their lives. There is a growing awareness and concern of the significant increase in learning disabilities in our children over the past 40 years. Autism, ADHD, dyslexia, mental retardation and many other learning and development disorders are currently prevalent and affect up to 15% of our children under the age of 18.[176]

Congenital infections (infections passed from the mom to the baby in utero or during birth), exposure to environmental chemicals, and prematurity are all major contributors to learning disabilities in children.[177]

Exposure to environmental chemicals begins even before a child is conceived and continues throughout its life. Young children are more susceptible to the adverse effects of chemical exposure. Children eat and breathe more than adults on a pound for pound basis so they are exposed to more toxins. The child's organ systems (especially the nervous system) are actively growing and are therefore more susceptible to the effects of chemicals. Young children put everything in their mouths, which is another source of exposure to chemical contaminants.[178]

Even very low doses of certain chemicals can alter gene expression, which impacts learning and development.[179]

Environmental agents that cause learning and developmental disabilities in humans
Alcohol
Lead
Mercury
PCBs
PBDEs
Manganese
Arsenic
Solvents
PAHs
Pesticides
Nicotine & environmental tobacco smoke

BEAUTY FROM WITHIN

We are just beginning to grasp the sheer magnitude of environmental chemicals and how they might impact our wellness. More people are choosing organic food and many are filtering their water. Yet we are resistant to reducing our chemical exposure when it affects our comfort and self-image.

The chemical assault begins as soon as we start our shower with unfiltered water. The skin is the largest organ of the body and chemicals from water are absorbed through the skin. To fully appreciate how well chemicals are absorbed through our skin, consider the birth control patch. This small patch on a woman's body delivers a set amount of hormone that is able to override and control her entire hormonal cycle. Or, how about the small nicotine patch that delivers enough nicotine through the skin to satisfy a smoker.

The chemical assault continues as we use our favorite shampoo and conditioner, shower gel, shaving cream, antiperspirant, hair straightening cream, hair mouse, gel, hair spray, peroxide and fluoride for our teeth (and all that other good stuff in our toothpaste), nail polish, makeup, perfume or cologne... you get my drift. Beauty has become an art and by the time we are ready for work we have literally lathered ourselves with a vast plethora of chemicals. Then we are off to the kitchen to get our fill of chemicals there.

Who can we blame for this one? Media and advertisers are likely candidates because they define beauty for us and entice us to try the endless treatments which promise to help us become more beautiful and therefore more happy. Women of all ages have bought into this façade. But as we aspire to reach the media's model of beauty, are we really happier? Is this good for us? I don't think so. We can never be perfect enough. Our boobs aren't big enough, our hips are too big, our legs are too short, our legs are too long, our nose is too long, our teeth aren't perfectly white, our hair is too straight, our hair is too curly, our hair is too thin, our complexion is not smooth enough, we have wrinkles, and the list goes on. Many women are so critical of their so-called inadequacies that they are willing to use whatever they can find to try to make themselves more beautiful, no matter how toxic the treatment. We must love ourselves enough to stop exposing ourselves to toxic treatments for the sake of beauty. As we focus on health, our natural beauty will shine through. We must make healthier choices.

Our awareness of the chemicals in our beauty products has grown in recent years. Parabins were considered a safe preservative and have been used for years in many beauty products. Several studies now show that parabins act as xenoestrogens (synthetic estrogens) in the body and have been found in breast tissue and in breast cancer tumors.

As we choose the lifestyle of a Wellness Champion building the Four Pillars of Wellness, we will reach our perfect body shape and will notice our natural beauty intensify. People will comment that we look younger and have a radiant glow. I have seen this exciting transformation many times in my clients. This is very empowering and allows us to not only accept ourselves but to really feel good about ourselves. Many women no longer feel that they need to wear foundation makeup because their skin complexion improves so much. Their hair and nails begin to grow. Women no longer have to hide behind all the stuff. Sure a little stuff that is free of harmful chemicals is fine, but it all comes down to balance, feeling and looking great, accepting who we are and having a great natural self-image.

PROCESSED FOODS—HIDDEN CHEMICALS

Companies that manufacture processed foods have one goal in mind: produce cheap calories that taste good and appeal to a multitude of consumers. Health will not be part of the equation until we demand it.

Processing foods often introduces chemicals into the finished product and thus toxins are found in unsuspected foods.

Dr. David Wallinga et al reported that many common foods containing high fructose corn syrup (HFCS) have unacceptable levels of mercury.[180]

HFCS is a common sweetener used in many processed foods such as soups, condiments, yogurts, breads, sandwich meats, granola bars, cereals and many beverages such as soft drinks. Many of these items are marketed to children.

For decades HFCS has been manufactured by using mercury-grade caustic soda. This study found mercury contamination in nearly one third of the 55 HFCS containing foods that it tested—from well-known brand names such as Quaker, Hunt's, Manwich, Hershey, Smuckers, Kraft, Nutri-Grain and Yoplait. The highest levels of mercury were detected in HFCS-containing dairy products, followed by salad dressings and condiments, and then snacks and desserts. Regulators who set safe fish consumption recommendations to prevent consumers from ingesting unsafe levels of mercury found in mercury-contaminated fish did not take into account the mercury found in HFCS foods. Other common household products such as shampoo, toilet tissue, bleach, and toothpaste are made from caustic soda and may also be contaminated with unacceptable levels of mercury.

The first step in reducing our exposure to toxins is to become aware of the multitude of toxins in our environment. We must then start making different choices. Remember to eat food that is as close to its natural or original state as possible. Avoid processed foods, especially HFCS.

ALCOHOL USE & ABUSE

We have had a love-hate relationship with alcohol throughout the ages. A nice glass of wine with a good meal or a cold beer on a hot day hits the spot. If we are healthy and do not have a history of dysbiosis, and alcohol is consumed in moderation, it won't have a major negative impact on our health. But all too often the consumption of alcohol is excessive, which causes economic, social, and personal hardships.

Alcohol is a mildly addictive drug and carcinogen that the liver must break down. Alcohol acts as a depressant. Drinking alcohol increases the risk of mouth, esophagus, pharynx, larynx and liver cancer in men and women, and breast cancer in women.[181]

Alcohol consumption trends dropped between the years 1990 –

1995 but then increased between the years 1995–2006.[182] Many individuals start drinking by the age of 13–14 years and those aged 18–25 years consume more alcohol than any other age group.[183]

I personally know people who buy organic food, take nutritional supplements, exercise, and basically follow the Initial Phase of the Candida program only to go out and become plastered on the weekend. Because they drink often, they must consume more alcohol than the average person just to get the alcohol buzz. Some of these individuals have serious health issues which likely stem from dysbiosis or silent infections. It saddens me to see that even though these people know that excessive alcohol consumption will place an additional burden on their body and will worsen their health, they can't control their consumption.

Alcohol is a toxin—a mycotoxin to be exact. It is a poison produced by yeast during fermentation. If you suspect that you have yeast/fungal overgrowth, then your body is already taxed with yeast toxins. Adding large amounts of alcohol will further compromise your health. If you are trying to re-establish balance in the GI tract, you must avoid alcohol for the short term. Your liver will be busy enough dealing with the toxins produced by the silent infections.

Alcoholism can sneak up on the best of us. If you chose to be a Wellness Champion but find yourself drinking often and/or many drinks at one time, you must ask yourself why you are doing this when you know that it is harmful to your health. Why are you often in an altered state when socializing? Is it a crutch? Why can't you go out and have fun being you. Some of you may be thinking "Of course I'm in control. I have a few drinks because I choose to. I could choose not too just as easily." If this is you, I challenge you to completely give up alcohol for one year and then re-evaluate. You may find it very liberating to be out with your friends, have a great time and feel refreshed the next day instead of tired and hung-over!

HOW TOXINS AFFECT US

It is virtually impossible to escape exposure to all synthetic chemicals.

They are present in the air we breathe, water we drink, clothes we wear, food we eat, personal care items we use, cleaners, beds, carpets, paints and the list goes on. Even though it may seem a daunting task, it is important to be aware of the constant bombardment of chemicals in our lives and make new choices that minimize our exposure to them.

Only in the past 10 years has science begun to understand some of the many ways that synthetic chemicals affect human health. It is not only the effect of each chemical that is a concern but also the combined or additive effect of several chemicals together. As you will see, many of these chemicals act as endocrine disrupters, immune suppressants, and carcinogens.

XENOESTROGENS

The endocrine system is made up of glands that manufacture precise amounts of specific hormones which regulate our mood, growth and development, as well as tissue function and metabolism. A healthy endocrine system supports abundant energy, the ability to handle stress, a restful uninterrupted sleep, mental alertness, healthy hair, skin, strong bones, balanced blood sugars, a healthy sex drive, optimal thyroid function, and the absence of PMS or menopausal symptoms. Therefore, a disruption in hormonal regulation can have a major impact on our quality of life.

Many synthetic chemicals act as xenoestrogens (manmade estrogens) in the body and disrupt normal hormonal regulation. Xenoestrogens are found in plastics, detergents, pesticides, petroleum products and beauty products, just to name a few. In the past, researchers felt that because xenoestrogens were present in small amounts they wouldn't affect our hormonal regulation. Researchers also dismissed concerns because they felt that the human estrogen hormone was much too strong for xenoestrogens to have an effect. Improved testing methods have proven these theories wrong.

Researchers found that combining 11 xenoestrogens in concentrations low enough that they would not show an effect on their own, led to a dramatic enhancement of the action of estrogen.[184] This study confirmed that xenoestrogens have an additive effect. If xenoestrogens are present alone and in a low enough concentration, they may not affect our hormonal system, but when combined with xenoestrogens from several sources their combined concentration can be detrimental to our hormonal system.

Our water sources have been contaminated by xenoestrogens for years. Consider all the pesticide residues, industrial wastes, synthetic hormones from both birth control pills and hormone replacement therapies, and the synthetic hormones and antibiotics used in agriculture, many of which find their way into our rivers, streams and lakes. It is no wonder that many of our fish are suffering with gender confusion.

GENDER CONFUSION IN OUR FISH

Several studies have raised concern about the emergence of gender confusion in fish. In 2004 researchers in Colorado tested three rivers—all downstream from sewage treatment plants—and found that male fish were developing female sexual organs due to estrogen and xenoestrogens present in the water. Female suckers outnumbered males 5 to 1 and 50% of the male fish had female sex tissue. Government officials noted that estrogen and xenoestrogen chemicals were present in 80% of the streams located in 30 American states.[185]

A Canadian study reported that estrogen-like contaminants in two Alberta rivers were seriously impacting the gender of the fish population.[186] It is typical to see about 55%–60% female gender, but in some stretches of the Old Man River they are observing up to 90% females.[187] They feel that the gender blending observed in these fish is due to the estrogen and xenoestrogen chemicals and they question whether this water is safe for humans to drink.[188]

This strong presence of estrogen and xenoestrogen in our water and environment is a real concern. One can't help but wonder how high levels of synthetic estrogens and xenoestrogens might affect the development of our children, especially in their early years.

MERCURY

Mercury is one of the most dangerous environmental toxins. It persists in our soil and water, and builds up in our tissues over time. Mercury is a neurotoxin and is extremely harmful to the development of the brain and nervous system in fetuses, infants and children.

Sources of mercury include contaminated seafood, amalgam fillings, vaccines, thermometers, HID lamps, batteries, preservatives, and pigments. Many processed foods containing high fructose corn syrup show levels of mercury.[189] Coal contains mercury and coal burning power plants in the U.S. are the largest source of human-caused mercury emission in that country. Approximately 25% of these emissions remain at home while the other 75% move into the global environment.[190]

Table 9. Possible symptoms of mercury exposure [191]

Possible Symptoms of Mercury Exposure
• Impaired peripheral vision
• Pins and needles feeling usually in the hands, feet, and around the mouth
• Skin rashes and dermatitis
• A lack of coordination of movements
• Impaired speech, hearing, walking
• Tremors
• Emotional changes (e.g. mood swings, irritability, nervousness, excessive shyness)
• Insomnia
• Headaches
• Changes in nerve responses
• Performance deficits on tests of cognitive function
• At higher exposures there may be kidney effects, respiratory failure and death
• Neuromuscular changes (such as weakness, muscle atrophy, twitching)
• Mental disturbances

* If you believe that you may have mercury poisoning see your medical doctor

In 2010, the U.S. Environmental Protection Agency reported that adults, children, and fetuses are at risk of mercury poisoning from contaminated sea food.[192] Pregnant women should avoid eating certain seafood that is contaminated with high levels of mercury and other toxins during pregnancy because the fetus is more vulnerable to mercury exposure than adults. Mercury can easily pass through the placenta[193] to the fetus. It is also important to check that your omega-3 fish oil supplement has been molecularly distilled to remove mercury and other heavy metals and toxins.

Amalgam fillings

Amalgam fillings are a significant contributor of mercury contamination due to the fact that approximately 40-50% of an amalgam filling is made of mercury.[194] Health Canada reported that amalgam fillings are the single largest source of mercury exposure for the average Canadian,[195] and that mercury is found in both our saliva and feces.[196] Mercury is released from amalgam fillings in our mouths as we chew our food. Many people have reported improvements to their health after their amalgam fillings were replaced with other alternatives such as white composite. If you decide to have your amalgam fillings removed it is important to work with a dentist who is very cautious and ensures that you don't swallow any of the filling during the process. As amalgam fillings are removed, toxic mercury vapors are released. Where women are concerned, do not have your amalgam fillings removed during pregnancy as you may be exposed to higher levels of mercury during the removal. Be sure to discuss these and any other concerns with your dentist before having this procedure done.

In January 2008, Norway, Sweden and Denmark banned the use of mercury in all dental care. These countries believe that there are satisfactory alternatives to amalgam that are less toxic to humans and do not have such a negative impact on our environment. Amalgam waste is the biggest source of mercury contamination in European Union (EU) waste water. Cremation also releases significant amounts of mercury into the atmosphere. In fact, dental amalgam and mercury from lab and medical devices accounts for 53% of the total mercury emissions in the UK and at least 7.4 tons of mercury are released into the water, atmosphere or land each year.[197] These countries believe that not using mercury in dental care will greatly reduce mercury pollution.

While other countries are banning the use of amalgam fillings, the FDA has decided that amalgam fillings are completely safe for adults and children. It seems very odd that the FDA is so accepting of amalgam.

The EPA on the other hand is concerned about the environmental impact of amalgam waste reaching the water supply. In 2003, the organization estimated that amalgam waste accounted for 50% of all mercury pollution in publicly-owned treatment works (POTWs).[198] In 2008, they estimated that every year about 160,000 dentists discharge about 3.7 tons of dental amalgam into the POTWs.[199] By 2012, the EPA plans to have a ruling in place that ensures that dentists reduce their amalgam waste by up to 95% by using amalgam separators.[200]

ENVIRONMENTAL TOXINS AND THE IMMUNE SYSTEM

Large databases of animal studies have shown that environmental chemicals suppress the immune system.[201] For example, numerous mammal studies have shown that dioxin suppresses the immune system.[202] Organotin is found in agricultural pesticides and is known to disrupt the endocrine system (interferes with our hormonal system). It also enhances allergic reactions and affects immune function.[203] Both environmental and occupational exposure to heavy metals is associated with allergy and autoimmune disease.[204]

In the past, experts could only go by individual case reports of people who experienced immune suppression after being exposed to chemicals on the job or by accident. Growing evidence implies that specific environmental chemicals modify normal immune reactions and cause disease progression in humans also.[205]

Cancer

Because people are exposed to so many chemicals at one time, it is challenging for researchers to determine if a particular chemical causes cancer. Nonetheless, research shows that exposure to certain synthetic chemicals increases the risk of various cancers in adults, especially cancers of the reproductive organs. For instance, endocrine disrupters play an important role in breast cancer[206] and prostate cancer.[207] In addition, mixtures of chemicals increase the risk of cancer.

Childhood cancer has been on the rise for years and researchers estimate that environmental factors could account for up to 90% of these cancers, depending on the type. Researchers Tami Gouveia-Vigeant and Joel Tickner reported the following:[208]

- Studies have consistently shown that children are more likely to develop certain childhood cancers if they or their parents were exposed to pesticides or solvents.
- Children with leukemia were 11 times more likely to have mothers who were exposed to pesticide sprays or foggers during pregnancy compared to healthy children.
- Children with fathers who were exposed to benzene and alcohols used in industrial products were 6 times more likely to develop leukemia if the exposure occurred before pregnancy compared to healthy children.
- Children who drank industrial contaminated well water were 5.4 times more likely to develop leukemia compared to healthy children.

The American Cancer Society's report *National Toxicology Program 11th Report on Carcinogens* lists more than 300 known and probable human carcinogens. Research in this area will continue to receive attention as cancer rates continue to rise and as better testing methods are available to measure the impact of environmental chemical exposure on humans.

CHILDREN: HOW TOXINS AFFECT LEARNING
& DEVELOPMENTAL DISORDERS IN OUR YOUNG

While the true cause of attention deficit hyperactivity disorder (ADHD) has not been determined, studies have linked ADHD to food additives and pesticides. A Harvard study found that children with ADHD had significantly higher levels of urinary pesticide metabolites than other children.[209] These findings confirm that current levels of pesticide residues in our food and environment may play a role in the prevalence of ADHD in children.

Mercury is an extremely toxic heavy metal that can harm the development of the brain and nervous system in fetuses, infants and children. Research shows that significant levels of mercury vapor can accumulate in the tissue of the fetus[210] and further research suggests that children who were exposed to mercury in the womb have lower neurodevelopment[211] which means that the growth and development of the brain in the area of emotions, learning ability and memory have been impaired.

Children exposed to mercury in the womb have also shown impaired cognitive thinking, memory, attention, language, and fine motor and visual spatial skills.[212]

The heated debate as to whether there is a direct link between mercury found in vaccines and the increased incidence of autism continues. Autism now affects approximately 1 in every 99 children.[213]

Thimerosal, a mercury-containing preservative used in vaccines and other drugs was first introduced in vaccines in the 1930s. Pharmaceutical companies increased the amount of thimerosal in vaccines in 1989.[214] Also, the number of vaccination injections given to children increased from 11 injections before 1989 to 24 injections after 1989.[215]

The incidence of autism and other developmental disorders in children has increased significantly over the years. Thimerosal has been removed from or reduced to trace amounts in all vaccines for children 6 six years old and under.[216] The influenza vaccine still contains thimerosal. It is important that a mom having her child vaccinated ask if the specific vaccination contains thimerosal. Don't just assume that it doesn't.

Although the debate continues, Dr. Mary Catherine DeSoto and Dr. Robert T. Hitlan[217] reviewed 58 studies and found that 43 of the studies suggest a link was present between thimerosal in vaccines and the increased incidence of autism, while only 13 studies found no link. This clearly shows that the evidence favors a link between the use of thimerosal in vaccines and the increased incidence of autism in children. This debate has high stakes for children, parents and pharmaceutical companies. The controversy may have been tainted with science that is biased. Pharmaceutical companies have been well-known to offer significant financial support to research that does not support a link between thimerosal and autism.[218]

Because mercury is a known neurotoxin which has devastating effects on a fetus and young children in general, I believe that it is in the best interest of mothers to minimize their exposure to mercury before, during, and after pregnancy and to minimize their child's exposure to mercury and other toxic heavy metals as much as possible. If you have several amalgam fillings in your mouth you may want to have them removed safely. Discuss this with an experienced dentist. This should not be done just before pregnancy or during pregnancy, as an accidental exposure to vapors or amalgam waste could be harmful to the fetus. You can have the level of mercury in your body tested through saliva or hair analysis. To reduce your exposure to environmental mercury, avoid high fructose corn syrup, amalgam fillings, thimerosal in vaccines, and contaminated seafood. I believe that it is better to err on the side of caution when it comes to mercury exposure.

YOUR OWN PERSONAL CHEMICAL FACTORY

As we become more aware of the chemicals in our external environment, we are better able to make different choices to reduce our exposure to them. This is important, but most of us are not aware of an even bigger chemical threat, one that may live inside us.

You may wonder why you feel so lousy some or all of the time, why you are so tired, why you suffer with such pain, or why you feel depressed, forgetful, or spacey. These complaints can be the consequence of your very own chemical factory. Silent infections in the body produce acids, alcohols, and many other chemicals that make us feel lousy and interfere with how our body should function.

This section will focus on how yeast or fungal overgrowth makes us sick. This is important for a couple of reasons. Firstly, this will give you a better understanding of what is going on in your body. It is also my hope that this section will pique the interest of many health care professionals who will then study the subject further. As a growing number of health care professionals acknowledge that dysbiosis exists and then learn how to help their patients restore balance, many people will be helped and many others will never have to suffer with it to begin with.

Dysbiosis caused by silent infections is epidemic in North America. This situation is what it is. We must not waste time blaming others but instead focus our energy on restoring balance within our bodies and share this information with our family, friends and co-workers so they can become empowered to do the same.

At this time most doctors have not been presented with enough proof that fungal/yeast overgrowth causes disease in people who are not immune suppressed. I believe that there is sufficient proof in the scientific literature, but it has not been properly compiled and therefore has not been acknowledged by the medical community. If you ask your doctor whether you could be suffering with yeast or fungal overgrowth you will likely get one of two responses. The first response will likely be that yeast does not cause disease unless you are an immune suppressed individual who has cancer, AIDS, or someone who has undergone organ transplant, etc. The second response might be that they have heard of this *theory* but there is no proof and if someone did have a fungal infection they would be really sick.

You might try to convince your doctor that he/she is wrong, but I wouldn't recommend that approach. A better approach would be to let them know that it is very important to you and ask them if they would be open to reviewing a document that presents peer reviewed scientific research on this topic. Remember that they are extremely busy and they are not interested in information that is just hearsay. Dr. Alex Vasquez has written an excellent paper, *Reducing Pain and Inflammation Naturally,* that you can share with your physician.[219]

Dr. Vasquez is a writer, speaker, and researcher who has obtained three doctoral healthcare degrees in three unique disciplines: chiropractic, naturopathic medicine, and osteopathic medicine—all from American universities.[220] You can find this scientific paper online. Please encourage your doctor to read it.

Keep in mind that some doctors still might not be interested in working with you. If this is the case, you may decide to find one who will. If you have built a good relationship with your doctor, he or she will usually be open to your input (even though they may not be convinced), as long as they feel it is a safe approach. The key here is to be patient and respectful. Although you may be really frustrated that they don't understand, losing your cool or being disrespectful will only make matters worse.

For many of us, dysbiosis started long ago. Because of our sheer ignorance, together with a diet rich in processed carbs (which fueled the infection that caused the dysbiosis), the population of bad guys continued to thrive to a point where the amount of toxins that they produced began to affect our health. There are many different parasites that harm humans, each one producing a variety of toxins that can make us sick. If you are a science buff or a skeptic I recommend that you read Dr. Vasquez's article.[221] This article is quite technical but you will gain a new appreciation for the sheer magnitude of parasites that we are exposed to and how they can affect our health and quality of life.

I will focus on the toxins produced by the yeast Candida, to keep things simple and because most of us have dealt with or are dealing with some degree of yeast overgrowth. As mentioned in the chapter, Minimize Silent Infections, small amounts of Candida are found in a healthy GI tract and since most of us have been on antibiotics in the past, most of us have some degree of fungal overgrowth. Please keep in mind that we are addressing just one parasite. Even so, I believe that this is where it all begins for the vast majority of us.

Candida produces more than 70 different toxins.[222] Examples include many acids, alcohols, mycotoxins and other chemicals that directly affect our blood sugar levels, mood, clarity of mind, energy level, immune function, and various other aspects of our health. Many doctors and researchers refuse to consider that Candida is more than an opportunist or a nuisance unless someone is dealing with cancer or HIV. Those of us who have suffered with Candidiasis know that this is not so.

Awareness of systemic Candida infections has grown significantly over the past 20 years and fortunately, there is a growing body of research that shows that Candida overgrowth produces chemicals that are detrimental to our health.

One such chemical is ethanol.[223] Several studies have reported about individuals with Candidiasis who ate a hefty carbohydrate meal and later complained of abdominal pain, bloating, mental confusion and slurred speech... almost like they were drunk... and they actually were. Science has a very technical name for this: they call it "auto-brewery." These people had their very own personal brewery within their body. The yeast overgrowth produced so much ethanol alcohol from the carbohydrate fermentation that they were literally drunk.

"Autobrewery is a syndrome that describes patients who become repeatedly inebriated after the ingestion of food with a high carbohy-drate content in the presence of abnormal yeast and bacterial intestinal proliferation."[224]

Candida sufferers often complain of feeling as though they have a hangover. I used to refer to it as *feeling like I was hit by a truck*. Candida strains have been shown to be massive producers of acetal-dehyde,[225] a neurotoxin that is responsible for the *hangover* after a drunk. Acetaldehyde is 10-30 times more toxic to humans than alcohol.[226] Not only does Candida produce acetaldehyde, but our body will also metabolize the ethanol produced by Candida into acetaldehyde providing even more of this neurotoxin.

Candida has the ability to weaken our defense mechanisms by producing enzymes called proteinases, which destroy our body's antibodies. Think of these enzymes as ferocious little packmen that digest any protein in their path. They also reduce the ability of our immune cells or soldiers to fight infection caused by bacteria and other microbes[227] leaving us more susceptible to secondary infections, especially in the GI tract. As secondary infections become established, they bring with them a host of new toxic metabolites and chemicals which will make us even sicker. This alone can result in many health problems.

The proteinase enzymes produced by Candida also destroy fibronectin which is found on the lining of the GI tract and prevents various bad bugs from attaching to the lining of the GI tract. Inflammation occurs as these packmen enzymes inflict extensive damage to the infected tissues.[228] Inflammation along the GI tract can cause maldigestion, malabsorption and leaky gut where large undigested molecules pass through the lining of the GI tract into the blood stream.[229] I hope you are beginning to appreciate the domino-like escalation of consequences caused by these infections.

Candida grows in our body much like a plant. It sends out roots called hyphae that push through the lining of the GI tract and then travels through the blood to settle in the lungs, reproductive organs, skin, sinuses, pancreas, liver and many other locations. As the fungal growth moves to various parts of the body, the secretion of the proteinase enzymes continues. These enzymes make yeast more resistant to being killed by our immune cells, activate molecules that constrict blood vessels affecting blood pressure, and appear to activate a blood clotting mechanism.[230]

Table 10 below outlines just a few toxic chemicals that yeasts produce and how they affect us. You will notice that these chemicals have the ability to suppress our immune system, act as carcinogens, initiate an allergic response, cause pain, affect our nervous system and endocrine system, our muscles, and cause inflammation. It is important to remember that this list does not include all the toxins produced by yeast overgrowth. Also, remember that there are many strains of Candida, other fungi, and many other parasites (bacteria, mycoplasma, mycobacteria, flukes, etc.) that cause disease in humans. This is just the tip of the iceberg!

Table 10. Metabolites and toxins produced by Candida albicans

Yeast Metabolite	How they affect us	Reference
Gliotoxin (mycotoxin)	Suppresses the immune system	1. Sutton, Newcombe, Waring, & Mullbacher. 1994[231] 2. Shah, Glover, & Larsen. 1995[232] 3. Shah, & Larsen. 1991[233] 4. Waring, & Beaver. 1996[234]
Ethanol (alcohol)	Carcinogen	1. Kaji et al. 1984[235] 2. Jansson-Nettelbladt, Meurling, Petrini, & Sjölin. 1995[236]
Acetaldehyde	Carcinogen	1. Kurkivuori et al. 2007[237] 2. Mukherjee et al. 2006[238]
Phenethyl alcohol	Irritant	1. Ghosh, Kebaara, Atkin, & Nickerson. 2008[239]
Tryptophol (alcohol)	Possible cytotoxic, cytostatic, and genotoxic effects	1. Ghosh, Kebaara, Atkin, & Nickerson. 2008[240] 2. Kosalec, Safranic, Pepeljnjak, Bacun-Druzina, Ramic, & Kopjar. 2008[241]
IgA-destroying proteinase (an enzyme that destroys antibodies)	1. Suppresses the immune system— reduced ability to fight infection (ex. bacteria) 2. Destroys keratin and collagen 3. Enhances vasoconstriction and blood clotting	1. Kaminishi et al. 1995[242] 2. Douglas. 1988[243]
Yeast/fungal organic acids	May interfere with normal cellular function	1. Great Plains Laboratory Inc. 2011[244]

Prostaglandins	1. Constricting or tightening of the airways 2. Suppresses the immune system 3. Expands blood vessels	1. Noverr, Toews, & Huffnagle. 2002[245] 2. Noverr, Phare, Toews, Coffey, & Huffnagle. 2001[246]
Formaldehyde	1. Corrosion of the gastrointestinal tract 2. Inflammation and ulceration of the mouth, esophagus, and stomach. 3. Cancer	1. Sakai, Tani. 1987[247]
Leukotrienes	1. Involved with asthma 2. Worsen airflow obstruction 3. Increased secretion of mucus and buildup of mucus 4. Constricting or tightening of the airways 5. Inflammation	1. Noverr, Toews, Huffnagle. 2002[248]

COULD ALLERGIES BE CAUSED BY AN INFECTION?

I'm sure that you will find this next section very intriguing. Many people suffer with allergies, asthma and eczema and experts are telling us that allergies are on the rise.[249] Allergies affect about 40–50 million Americans[250] and 10 million Canadians.[251]

Between 1997 and 2007, food allergies in our children under the age of 18 increased by 18%.[252] Children with food allergies are two to four times more likely to suffer with asthma or eczema.[253]

Fungal or yeast overgrowth causes inflammation in the body and is intimately associated with allergic diseases, such as asthma, sinusitis, bronchpulmonary mycoses and hypersensitivity pneumonitis.[254] A study by researchers at the Mayo Clinic in 1999 tested over two hundred people with sinusitis and found that 96% of them tested positive for fungal growth. One hundred of these patients were treated with surgery and the researchers found fungal mucin and many white blood cells in 96% of these people.[255] Mucin is a mucous-type gel that our cells produce to trap pathogens like fungi and bacteria.

"Fungus allergy was thought to be involved in less than ten percent of cases," says Dr. David Sherris.[256] "Our studies indicate that, in fact, fungus is likely the cause of nearly all of these problems. And it is not an allergic reaction, but an immune reaction."

It is interesting that our cells produce an overabundance of mucin in both fungal sinus infections and also in many types of cancer. Could it be that the overproduction of mucin in chronic fungal sinusitis and in cancer are related or possibly have the same cause? Could the cause for both be an infection?

The Mayo researchers concluded that the patients in the study were not allergic to fungus but suffered with fungal growth in their sinuses. It is hard to believe that this study was done more over 10 years ago, and yet we are still carrying out the same ineffective treatments for sinusitis today.

Fungal growth also produces certain chemical messengers called prostaglandins and leukotrienes.[257] These hormone-like compounds are able to create very strong responses in the body and are potent immune system regulators. Our body makes these compounds at specific times and in specific amounts. Once these compounds have done their job they are quickly removed and excreted. They don't just hang around because the response that they elicit in the body is too powerful.

The presence of prostaglandins in our airways causes the airways to constrict or tighten and our blood vessels to open. Leukotrienes are involved with asthma as they cause or worsen airflow obstruction, increase mucus secretion and the buildup of mucus, constrict the airways, and cause an inflammatory response. Leukotrienes protect the body against attacks from invaders and are also part of the allergic response.

The body is a miracle. It is genetically programmed to know precisely how to operate. If we do not know the cause of allergies, how can we assume that the body is so stupid that it would produce leukotrienes and thus inflammation for no good reason? The body is not stupid!

It makes more sense that either the body is producing these chemicals in response to a silent infection in the airways of the lungs, or maybe a silent infection is directly producing the leukotriene chemicals causing the inflammatory response. It is interesting that leukotriene receptor antagonist (LTRAs) medications are used to treat asthma. They block leukotrienes that are causing the inflammation. So instead of determining why leukotrienes are present when they normally shouldn't be, we assume that the body is stupid and we use a drug to block the action of the leukotrienes; instead of determining what is interfering with the body's ability to operate optimally, we mask the problem with a band-aid. We treat the symptom and do not address the cause and thus over time the condition usually progresses and general health deteriorates. It has been my observation that as silent infections are minimized in the body, the immune system is strengthened and balance is restored through the Four Pillars of Wellness, leukotrienes are no longer produced and the symptoms of asthma diminish.

The Asthma Society of Canada's website states that "inhaled steroids are generally considered to be the best option... for asthma control."[258] If fungal overgrowth is involved in asthma and may even be a cause of asthma, it is unfortunate that inhaled corticosteroids—one of the main treatments for asthma—has as one of its main side effects thrush or yeast overgrowth in the mouth.[259] Steroids directly enhance the growth of fungi and yeast by suppressing the immune system and causing an increase in blood sugar.[260] It is ironic that the most popular treatment for asthma may be exacerbating the fungal infection, making the cause of the asthma worse.

We know that fungal overgrowth produces compounds that bring about allergy and asthma symptoms in people. We also know that many doctors believe that allergies, asthma and eczema are intimately associated with fungal growth. So is it possible that the underlying cause of allergy, asthma and eczema is a fungal or yeast infection?

You be the judge. Once again, common sense goes a long way. I can hear the skeptics "This has not been accepted by main stream medicine!" My response to that would be, "go ahead and wait for it to be accepted. You may have to wait a very long time considering that this group doesn't believe that yeast and fungal overgrowth is a problem to begin with."

If you have many symptoms of a fungal infection, try the program with the guidance of an experienced health care professional and see for yourself if you experience an improvement in your health. It can't hurt to try this approach, and it might very well change your life.

My life changed when I put my personal chemical factory out of business through building the Four Pillars of Wellness.

Dr. Vasquez sums it up nicely as he states, "Clinical experience has shown us again and again that eradicating dysbiosis helps normalize immune function, alleviate autoimmunity and allergy, reduce inflammation, improve detoxification, and to help 'cure' people of their previously 'incurable' multiple chemical sensitivity and environmental illness."[261]

Beware

At this time most health care professionals—even complementary providers do not fully grasp the full extent to which dysbiosis affects our health. Any medical professional that does understand the challenge at hand will be hard to find as they work quietly so as not to draw attention to themselves for fear of being ostracized by their peers. This is improving in larger cities.

Time and time again health care professionals have assured me that they understand the serious nature of silent infections and yet still take my clients down bunny trails dealing with emotions, adrenal support, hormone therapy, food desensitization, etc., without first aggressively treating the silent infection. These clients spend hundreds or thousands of dollars on various therapies and do not see major improvements until the infection is dealt with.

The vast majority of the population in North America has taken antibiotics in the past and is therefore dealing with some degree of dysbiosis. There are just too many of us that suffer with dysbiosis to blame it on our emotions or a suppressed immune system. When we suffer with dysbiosis, we don't handle stress as well because our body is already taxed from the infection. The chemicals produced by the infection can affect our thinking and mood, cause allergies, tax our adrenals and other glands and organs, and suppress our immune system. It is extremely important to get to the root cause of all the symptoms or complaints and in my experience the best approach is to first address the silent infection aggressively. Once balance in the GI tract is restored, the chemical toxins of the infection are eliminated, and nutritional deficiencies from the infection are corrected, disease symptoms often cease and desist almost miraculously.

Pillar #4
Build A Healthy Lifestyle

ARE YOU RUNNING YOUR LIFE OR IS LIFE RUNNING YOU?

Our beliefs around lifestyle and our daily habits affect our quality of life in more ways than we realize. Lifestyle is the fourth pillar of wellness and includes getting our beauty sleep, soaking up a healthy amount of sunshine, having fun, getting active, and nurturing our soul. This is what many would consider the holistic pillar of wellness because it impacts our emotional, mental, spiritual, and physical wellness. This section is like the icing on the wellness cake. Building this pillar makes the difference between a mediocre life and a life of purpose, passion and design.

YOUR BEAUTY SLEEP

Getting enough sleep is important for optimal brain, cardiovascular system and immune function. Adequate sleep improves our memory, insight and ability to learn. We learn new skills better when we are well rested and we remember what we've learned better if we have a good night's sleep.

Benefits of a good night's sleep include (7–8 hours … or more if needed):[262]

- The brain's thinking processes operate faster
- Increased ability to focus
- Improved decision making, creativity, and ability to learn
- Improved memory
- Shorter reaction time
- Improved mood—happy vs. irritable
- Decreased risk of obesity. During sleep the body produces more of the appetite suppressant hormone leptin and less of the appetite stimulant hormone ghrelin.
- Decreased risk of diabetes.
- Improved cardiovascular health
- Improved immune function
- Improved ability to fight infections
- Quicker muscle recovery
- Optimal growth in children
- Decreased risk of depression
- Improved fertility in women

Sleep is a powerful regulator of appetite, energy use and weight control. Studies show that people who get about 5 hours of sleep each night are much more likely to become obese than people who get 7–8 hours of sleep each night.[263]

How much sleep do I need?

The amount of sleep that we need varies from one person to the next. Different age groups also tend to need different amounts of sleep. Generally, adults need 7–8 hours of sleep each night while newborns need 16–18 hours, preschoolers need 10–12 hours each night and adolescents require at least 9 hours.[264] Although seniors often have a hard time falling asleep and/or wake up early in the morning and/or are awake for hours in the middle of the night, there is no research to support the idea that the elderly need less sleep than adults in general. These disruptions in sleep are mostly caused by illness or they are side effects of the medications that they are taking.[265]

Sleep disruptors

- Stimulants—caffeine [found in soft drinks, coffee or tea], nicotine
- Alcohol
- Pharmaceuticals—decongestants, steroids, beta blockers, many pain relievers, asthma medication
- Conditions such as depression, schizophrenia, bipolar, and anxiety disorders cause insomnia
- Psychological stress
- Hormonal imbalances

Tips for getting a great night's sleep

- Build the Four Pillars of Wellness—maximize nutrition, minimize silent infections, reduce exposure to toxins, and optimize your lifestyle
- Make an effort to go to bed at the same time each night
- Have your last meal several hours before bed

- Exercise during the day (not before bed)
- Get at least 30 min. of sunlight exposure each day
- If you are having sleeping difficulties, avoid all stimulants
- Make sure that your bedroom is dark and quiet while you sleep
- Open your window slightly while you sleep to bring in fresh cool air
- If you live on a noisy street you can run an air filter fan in your bedroom during the night. The steady hum of the fan will drown out the erratic sounds of the traffic.
- Drink chamomile tea
- Read for a few minutes before bed or listen to soft music. Turn down the main lights and grab a good book and nurture your soul.
- Deep breathing. Close your eyes and slowly take a deep breath pushing out your belly, hold it for a few seconds and then slowly breathe out as much air as you can. With the next breath try to breath in deeper and make your exhale longer than your inhale.
- Muscle relaxation. As you are lying in bed completely relaxed tense up your toes, hold for 10 seconds and then relax. Continue to tense, hold and then relax each muscle of your body moving up from your toes to your head.
- Focus your mind on something that you find really relaxing or peaceful. If I am overstimulated or my mind is racing I can settle it down by focusing on a time that I was lying on a beach at the ocean. I focus on the warmth of the sun, the sounds of the waves and how relaxed I felt at that time. Next thing I know... it's morning.

Insomnia

If you have been in bed for a while and you are becoming anxious, it is better to take your mind off this by reading or do a relaxation activity rather than to just lay there and become more anxious. A snoring partner can also make it difficult for someone to fall asleep or remain sleeping.

Most of us have suffered with insomnia at some point in our lives.

It's not a major concern if occasionally you can't fall asleep, or you wake up in the middle of the night for an hour or two. But if this occurs several times a week for a month or more you should pay attention. First, follow the tips listed on page 183. This will most often get the sleeping pattern back on track.

If you have suffered with insomnia for some time, make sure to visit your health care provider. If your doctor has ruled out all possible medical concerns, they may suggest a sleep aid which can be helpful if you haven't slept well for a long time. A sleep aid can help break this cycle. Natural sleep aids such as valerian root or melatonin can be very effective. Nonprescription pharmaceuticals can also be a big help. The body will become dependent on prescription pharmaceutical sleeping pills. Always work with a health care provider to find a safe and effective sleep aid. The goal is to use the sleep aid for a short period of time, not to use it as a crutch.

GET ACTIVE!

If it is common knowledge that exercise is such an important part of wellness, why do so many of us avoid it? We complain that we are too busy, too tired, or it's too cold, hot or wet outside.

The biggest barrier to physical activity is lack of time, or is it that lack of time is our most common excuse? I believe that our lack of consistent activity is the result of beliefs that we hold, beliefs that do not value the importance of physical activity. Beliefs such as:

- I can't exercise in the winter because I hate the cold
- I can't afford a gym membership
- I am just too busy
- I am way too tired
- I am healthy. I don't need to exercise
- I can't exercise because I …

If we truly believed that our life depended on us staying active, most of us would make sure to fit it into our busy schedules. Also, if exercise was actually fun, we would more likely commit to making it a regular part of our lives. Physical activity must be part of our lifestyle pillar of wellness plan because it:[266]

- Promotes a longer life and better quality of life
- Improves our energy level
- Improves brain function
- Improves immune function
- Improves our mood by stimulating chemicals in the brain that make us feel happier and more relaxed after the activity
- Helps prevent depression
- Makes us look and feel better, improving our self-esteem and self confidence
- Is important in the prevention and management of high blood pressure
- Reduces our risk of chronic diseases such as type 2 diabetes, osteoporosis and certain types of cancer
- Improves cardiovascular health—boosts the good cholesterol while decreasing triglycerides, and reduces plaque build-up in the arteries
- Helps us to maintain our perfect body shape
- Improves circulation and the delivery of oxygen and nutrients to tissues
- Improves sleep—we fall asleep quicker and experience a deeper sleep which translates to better mood, concentration, and productivity during the day
- Improves our sex life
- Can be loads of fun

If you have medical concerns make sure you consult with your doctor about any activities that you would like to start. Also, if you are under a significant amount of stress, it may be wise to decrease the intensity of the exercise activity until the stressful period passes. Being active will offset the effects of stress, but you may choose walking instead of running during the really stressful time.

Exercise stresses the body, albeit this is good stress. If you are under significant stress (personal, financial, emotional, or sickness, etc.) choosing a lower impact activity will still provide the benefits of exercise without taxing the body when it is already taxed to the max. Listen to your body. Pay attention to how you feel and choose activities accordingly.

How to make exercise more fun:

1. **Have fun.** Pick an activity or activities that you really enjoy. Don't exercise for the sake of exercise, but book fun time for yourself and pick an activity that makes you happy!

2. **Find an exercise buddy.** Pick someone who is positive, fun and committed to wellness; someone you love to spend time with and someone who will cheer you on and hold you accountable to your goals.

3. **Join a group fitness class or group.** Choose a group or class that you think will be fun. If you try it for a month or two and find that you don't enjoy it, try something else and don't stop until you find activities that you can't wait to do. It can be a great opportunity to make new friends. The options are endless. If you like the outdoors, some examples include hiking, walking, running, biking or Nordic (pole) walking groups. In a gym setting you will find spin, Pilates, martial arts, dance, yoga, Tae Bo, and skipping classes. Dance classes have come a long way. Fitness facilities offer hip-hop, ballet, African, zumba, choreography, broadway and cabaret, belly, Latino and ballroom just to name a few. Public swimming facilities offer aquafit classes, and rock wall climbing has also become very popular. Instructors can be inspiring, motivating and challenge you to play full out and reap the many benefits of physical fitness.

4. **Join a team.** There are volleyball, basketball, hockey, soccer, softball, tennis, golf, and many other city leagues. Find a sport that you enjoyed and were good at in your younger years or try a new sport.

Team sports are a great way to build friendships while getting fit.

5. **Multitask.** Multitasking is not always effective, but here it can work. Nurture your soul by listening to your favorite inspirational music if you are doing a cardio and/or resistance routine at home or outdoors. Download professional development or inspirational presentations, audio books, or podcasts onto your favorite media player (MP3 or iPod). This will allow you to learn something new or nurture your soul while you are getting active.

6. **Mix it up and challenge yourself.** If you are easily bored, make sure to include a good variety of activities. If you find that the activities have become routine, it's time to mix it up.

7. **Throw out the scale: measure don't weigh.** If you are not at your ideal body weight, and you want to track your progress it is okay to chart your measurements using a tape measure. Don't use a weight scale. Measure and chart the change in your upper arms, chest, stomach, waist, upper thighs and calves. Be careful to measure the same place each time. As you follow the Four Pillars of Wellness, you will burn and release fat while building muscle. Muscle weighs about 3 times more than the same amount of fat. If you step on a scale you may feel that your weight is not dropping as quickly as you would like, this is because you are burning fat and replacing it with lean muscle, which weighs more. If you measure your body, you will notice that you are losing inches of fat, and this will excite you!

8. **Make it a family affair.** One of the biggest challenges facing families today is that we are just too busy. This *busyness* has had an impact on the family unit. We as parents and spouses must be constantly aware of this and make sure that we are spending daily quality time with the important people in our lives. Hiking, biking, walking, playing a game of soccer, badminton, chasing our kids around the playground are just a few examples of activities that we can enjoy with our family. This precious, fun time builds relationships, keeps us active and will leave long-lasting memories with our loved ones.

Aerobic vs. Anaerobic (Cardio vs. Endurance)

Cardio activities increase heart rate, while endurance activities build and maintain muscle mass. Both types of activities are important. The American College of Sports Medicine (ACSM)[267] and the American Heart Association (AHA)[268] have outlined the following basic guidelines for healthy adults under age 65:

"Do moderately intense cardio activities 30 minutes each day, five days a week **or** do vigorously intense cardio 20 minutes each day, 3 days a week. And do eight to ten different strength-training exercises, (8 to 12 repetitions of each exercise) twice a week." This recommendation is for an average healthy adult who wants to maintain their health and reduce the risk of chronic illness. These are the minimum recommendations for a healthy adult under 65 years of age. If you can fit more activities into your day, go for it, you will benefit all the more.

Moderate-intensity physical activity means that you are active enough to raise your heart rate and sweat, but you can still carry on a conversation.

Time Savers

- Plan ahead—look at your weekly schedule and set aside specific times where you are able to fit activities in. Make exercise part of your daily schedule just as you do for everything that is important.
- Do activities at home, before or after work—saves driving time
- Get active during lunch
- Do activities in short bouts—two 15 min. or three 10 min. bouts of activity can be substituted for one 30 min. bout.

Exercise, cheap medicine

Getting active doesn't have to be expensive. It just takes some motivation and a good pair of running shoes. The rewards include lots of energy, a stronger immune system and a decreased risk of disease, all while you are having fun. The rewards of regular activity are too great to pass it by.

SUNSHINE

Sunshine has had its share of bad press over the years. Experts have warned us of the thinning ozone layer, higher levels of UV radiation, and our increased risk of cancer. It has come to the point where some parents won't allow their children to go outside unless they are completely covered with sunscreen or clothing. This is really unfortunate because there are many benefits to getting a healthy dose of daily sunshine.

Benefits of sunshine:
- Increases our body's supply of vitamin D
- Improved immune function
- Decreased risk of osteoporosis
- Optimal bone formation in children
- Down regulation of immune response—good for autoimmune diseases
- Reduces the risk of melanoma and other cancers[269, 270]
- Improvements in psoriasis
- Increased release of endorphin molecules which act as pain relievers and make us feel good

What blocks our body's ability to make vitamin D from sunshine?
- Clothing
- Excess body fat
- Sunscreen
- The skin pigment melanin

Sunshine has the ability to increase the body's supply of vitamin D. Caucasians produce about 50,000 IU of vitamin D in just 30 min. of sunbathing in a swimming suit on a sunny day. Tanned folks produce 20,000–30,000 IU and dark-skinned people produce 8,000–10,000 in the same 30 min. time period.[271]

Lack of sunlight leads to a deficiency of vitamin D, and experts feel that this deficiency is a major cause of poor health.[272] A report by the World Health Organization warns that although high levels of ultra violet radiation (UVR) from the sun is detrimental to our health, very low levels of UVR from the sun is likely responsible for an increase in disorders of the musculoskeletal system, and also certain autoimmune diseases and life threatening cancers.[273]

We have a problem. Current government agency guidelines recommend that people should minimize their exposure to sunlight especially during midday, which is actually the best time for vitamin D synthesis, especially in countries with less sunshine and colder temperatures. Our increasingly indoor lifestyle has also reduced our exposure to sunshine.

A growing number of researchers are concerned that strong efforts to keep the public from excessive UVR exposure is obscuring the many health-promoting benefits of sunlight. They believe that the benefits of moderate sun exposure far outweigh any adverse effects, and that any risks can be minimized by avoiding excessive UVR exposure (i.e. sunburns).[274]

Sunshine is a very important piece of the wellness puzzle. Get active outdoors whenever possible. The fresh air will be an added bonus to your activities. Enjoy the sunshine, but do so in moderation. Avoid getting sunburns and don't spend hours baking in the sun, even if you are lathered in sunscreen.

NURTURE YOUR SOUL

We are spiritual beings. We are aware of *self* while other animals are not, and we contemplate the afterlife. Humans feel a sense of right and wrong, good and evil. We are able to communicate and use our brains in much more complex ways than all other animals. We search for long-term relationships because we have a deep desire to love and be loved. We long to define our purpose in life.

Faith is an interesting concept. It can only happen when we believe in something without any physical proof. We can't prove it but we know that it is true because we have experienced it.

Most people believe that God exists and that we are spiritual beings. I appreciate and respect that we come from diverse faith backgrounds. I believe that nurturing our soul adds an incredible dimension to our happiness and wellness. Adding this component can make the difference between a mere physical existence and a life filled with passion and purpose, where our life and work becomes a mission.

I know that I would not have had the same level of success in reclaiming my health if I tried to figure all this out on my own. I leaned on God in my darkest times and had the comfort of knowing that he was always with me, answering my prayers and guiding me. He always brought the right information or people into my life at the right time. He has never allowed more on my plate than I could handle. There were times when I felt that I couldn't handle any more and he has always come through for me. Sometimes the answer would come in ways that I did not expect. All I know is that the more that I try to run my life on my own, the more things become messed up, and the more I include Him in my life the more amazing my life unfolds.

I am so grateful to have a second chance at enjoying an excellent quality of life and I am so blessed to play a small part in helping others improve their quality of life. God gives me tremendous inner strength, peace and joy. I give him all the credit for any success that I enjoy with respect to my health, marriage, three beautiful children and my mission in life.

I believe that it is very important to nurture your soul and I encourage you to practice your faith if you have one, or go back to the faith of your childhood. If you search for God, you will find him and your life will never be the same!

Women's Health Issues

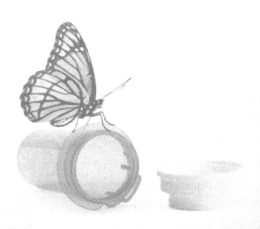

Yeasts plague women more than men—thanks to those hormones which give us our curvy shape, make us sensitive, loving and yes... emotional at times.

The monthly rise and fall of our sex hormones affects how our immune system functions and has an impact on our blood sugar levels. Silent infections in the body will prosper with higher blood sugar levels or when the immune system is modulated by hormones. As this bad crew prospers we suffer with intense cravings and hunger, bloating, mood issues, low blood sugar, as well as an increase in toxic chemicals circulating in our bodies.

I don't believe that strong premenstrual symptoms (PMS) or major menopausal symptoms should be a normal part of being a woman. In my own personal experience and in coaching many women, PMS symptoms and menopausal symptoms are most often the consequence of silent infections, nutrient deficiencies and toxic loads. As women build their Four Pillars of Wellness, pre-menstrual symptoms subside and one day they realize their period has arrived without the dreadful reminders from symptoms that used to appear a week or two before.

As silent infections are dealt with and nutritional deficiencies are corrected, cycles become regular, cramps are no longer an issue, women no longer feel like crying or tearing someone's head off days before their period, and heavy bleeding diminishes.

Silent infections, and especially Candida overgrowth, can really mess with a woman's quality of life. Here is a list of common complaints that can be caused by Candida overgrowth:

- PMS symptoms—intense cravings and or hunger, bloating, mood swings, irritability, anxiety, anger outbursts, depression, fatigue, headaches, and the list continues...
- Menopausal symptoms
- Cloudy white cottage cheese-like vaginal discharge
- Vaginal itch, or burning
- Heavy bleeding during the period
- Cramping during menstrual period

- Endometriosis
- Low blood iron (anemia) or low ferritin
- Breast cysts or lumpy breasts at certain times of the month
- Plugged milk ducts while breast feeding
- Cracked sore nipples
- Ovarian cysts
- Polycystic ovarian disease
- Cystitis

As young women reach puberty and sex hormone production increases, existing dysbiosis symptoms often worsen. Higher levels of the sex hormones are associated with reduced insulin sensitivity, higher blood sugar levels, suppression of immune function and higher levels of anti-Candida antibodies.[275,276,277]

A decrease in insulin sensitivity has been reported during the second half of the menstrual cycle leading up to menstruation,[278] which means that insulin is less effective at lowering blood sugar levels during this period of time. This can result in higher blood sugar levels, and more sugar in the blood means more food for yeast overgrowth. The body's precise regulation of blood sugar levels and immune function is important to support a future pregnancy. Silent infections will benefit from this.

This could help explain why many women notice an increase in digestive symptoms and almost half of women with irritable bowel syndrome report an increase in symptoms during the second half of the menstrual cycle leading up to the period.[279] PMS symptoms also escalate during this time.

One study measured anti-Candida antibodies in the blood of three groups of normal women who were free of clinical symptoms of Candidiasis. Women in the first group were in the first half of their menstrual cycle where estrogen is higher. The second group of women were in the second half of their menstrual cycle where progesterone is higher. And the third group of women were long time users of a birth control pill high in the synthetic progesterone hormone called progestin. The researchers found that women in the second half of the menstrual cycle had twice the number of anti-Candida antibodies as women in the first half of the menstrual cycle. Also, women who were long time users of the birth control pill high in synthetic progestin had three times the anti-Candida antibodies in their plasma.

Although the occurrence of increased digestive complaints and PMS are not well understood by science or medicine, it is likely that higher blood sugar levels and a down-regulated immune system due to changes in hormones encourage silent infections to prosper during this time, resulting in many of these undesirable symptoms. Higher levels of progesterone are associated with a down regulation of the inflammatory immune response,[280] while the drop in progesterone levels just before menstrual period results in an enhancement of inflammatory immune mediators.[281]

An increase in the growth of yeast or other silent infection in the week or two leading up to the menstrual period may also help explain why some women experience painful menstrual cramps caused by the production of prostaglandins. Prostaglandins are chemical messengers produced by the body; as they cause inflammation and pain, many women reach for painkillers.

Prostaglandins are produced by the body. High concentrations of prostaglandins are found in the endometrium (lining of the uterus). They are potent messenger molecules that have very specific functions. The big question is "Why is there an excessive production of prostaglandins in some women during the menstrual period?" Once again there are many hypotheses but no conclusive answers.

Researchers have demonstrated that although prostaglandins are produced by the body, they can also be produced directly by yeast (and other microbes), or by the body in response to an infection.[282] Many medical experts recommend that women who are prone to menstrual cramps take ibuprofen a few days before menstruation to block the production and action of prostaglandins. Taking pain medication may relieve immediate pain but does not address the cause of this condition.

The body is so sophisticated. It doesn't make sense that some women should suffer with menstrual cramps on a monthly basis. We must consider why prostaglandins are produced in excess. Pain is not a normal physiological response to having a menstrual period. What is interfering with the body's ability to function optimally? If the increased production of prostaglandins is the result of a silent infection, then just masking the symptoms and ignoring the infection will only allow it to gain more ground over time.

SAY GOODBYE TO PMS

Up to 85% of women suffer with at least one of the following premenstrual symptoms:[283] acne, swollen tender breasts, fatigue, insomnia, digestive issues, headaches, backaches, food cravings, ravenous hunger, joint or muscle pain, mood swings, irritability, depression, anxiety, or difficulty concentrating. That the vast majority of women experience some of these symptoms every month is torture and just plain ridiculous.

If the cause of PMS is not dealt with, new symptoms will continue to surface and general health will continue to decline. It's like putting a bandage on an abscess. The infection will continue to fester even though it has been covered up.

We must adopt a new philosophy; discover what is interfering with our body's ability to perform optimally and address it. For long term success we must adopt a holistic approach and build the Four Pillars of Wellness.

YEAST INFECTIONS

You may wonder which came first—the vaginal yeast infection or yeast overgrowth in the GI tract. As we take broad spectrum antibiotics, our natural defense in the GI tract is destroyed but this is also true for other parts of the body such as our sinuses, respiratory tract, and parts of our genitourinary system,[284] so in a way it doesn't really matter what came first.

Many women are treated repeatedly for vaginal yeast infections and wonder why they keep getting the infection back or why they continue to have a low grade vaginal infection. There are several reasons for this. Candida causes inflammation as it damages the tissue it infects. It also produces the toxin gliotoxin which suppresses the immune system,[285] and Candida directly destroys our antibodies that fight yeast. All this together is believed to cause the immune system to become sensitized toward allergy and pro-inflammatory disease.[286] The medical community believes that Candida and other yeast infections only cause disease in individuals who have a suppressed immune system... but in fact yeast overgrowth suppresses the immune system.

Dr. Paula Moraes et al reported that women with chronic yeast overgrowth in the GI tract were nearly two times more likely to suffer with hay fever (allergic rhinitis) than women who did not have yeast overgrowth.[287]

The results of a study by Dr. Mary Rylan Miles et al[288] found that if Candida albicans was cultured from the vagina it was always found in the stool, and conversely that if it was not isolated from the stool it was never found in the vagina. These researchers concluded that women with chronic vaginal yeast overgrowth always have yeast overgrowth in the GI tract and that in order to successfully permanently cure the vaginal yeast infection, the reservoir of yeast overgrowth in the GI tract had to be treated also.

A woman can have a low grade vaginal infection and not be aware of it. This was my experience for many years. Many women will suffer with the classic symptoms of a vaginal yeast infection which include severe itching and burning, but many other women never have these symptoms and therefore don't realize that they have a low grade vaginal yeast infection. Your only symptoms may be an occasional small amount of opaque white discharge.

So how do you know if you have a vaginal yeast infection?

Your best bet is to go by symptoms. If you answered yes to one or more of the first five questions in the Diagnosing Fungal Overgrowth survey (page 110) and you checked some of the symptoms in the Common Symptoms of Chronic Yeast Overgrowth (page 112) and you have noticed a white opaque vaginal discharge during the month, chances are you do have a vaginal yeast infection. If this is the case your best long term success will come from restoring balance to the GI tract while you treat the vaginal yeast infection, and once again by building the Four Pillars of Wellness. Work with an experienced health care professional to establish a program that works.

PREGNANCY WELLNESS

Because silent infections are linked with miscarriages and premature labor and birth, it is vital that women who wish to start a family minimize silent infections and optimize their wellness before they become pregnant. Pregnancy taxes the female body and it is important that a woman goes into pregnancy strong and healthy for her sake and the sake of her baby.

It is well established that yeast infections are common in pregnancy.[289] This is not to infer that pregnancy causes vaginal yeast infections, but rather if a woman has a history of yeast overgrowth, pregnancy will often exacerbate it. Although medicine does not fully understand why this is so, research is providing clues that help explain this phenomenon. During pregnancy women experience a down-regulation of the immune response[290] and an increased amount of glucose (sugar) in the blood, both of which can promote yeast overgrowth.

It is remarkable how the immune system of a pregnant woman accepts the developing baby. The fetus is foreign tissue and a normal immune response would be to destroy the foreign tissue. The woman's body not only accepts the fetus but her body also adapts to the growing nutritional needs of her developing child.

How the immune system of an expectant mom adapts to accept

the fetus is complex and not well understood.[291] The innate immune response defends us from infection in an immediate way, and in general terms it is accepted that pregnancy is associated with a shift away from inflammatory immune responses toward anti-inflammatory immune responses.[292]

Regulatory T (Treg) cells are an example of this as they are potent suppressors of both autoimmunity and organ transplant rejection. These immune cells protect our tissues from overactive immune responses. Pregnant women have an increased number of Treg cells vs. non-pregnant women. Treg cells may protect the fetus from the pregnant mom's normal immune response to foreign tissue. Expectant women who have deficiencies in Treg cells are linked with infertility and miscarriage.[293]

The presence of increased numbers of Treg cells in pregnant women may help to explain why pregnant women with autoimmune disease experience a reduction in autoimmune symptoms during pregnancy.

We have discussed that silent infections and in particular, yeast overgrowth are intimately linked with and are likely a cause of autoimmune disease. Also, inflammation is the body's response to infection or damage. If this is the case, then a down-regulated immune system in a pregnant woman with a history of autoimmune disease would allow any existing yeast overgrowth to benefit. The silent infection causing the autoimmune response is still present in the pregnant woman, but during the pregnancy the immune system may not fight it as aggressively because the inflammatory processes are suppressed to protect the developing baby.

Researchers have also observed that high levels of the molecule MIC-1 in pregnant women modulate inflammation by suppressing molecules that cause inflammation.[294]

We have considered just two ways that a pregnant woman's immune system adapts in order to accept the implantation and the presence of a developing child. In both cases, inflammatory immune responses are suppressed. Therefore if inflammation is present before pregnancy, due to the presence of silent infections it makes sense that these modifications to the immune response during pregnancy could benefit a silent infection.

Glucose production during pregnancy

As the fetus grows it requires more glucose, and studies show that the rate of appearance of glucose in the expectant mom's blood is significantly higher in the first, second, and third trimester of pregnancy than in non-pregnant women. Insulin causes cells to take up glucose from the blood, thus lowering blood sugar levels. The action of insulin is lower in pregnant woman vs. non-pregnant women. In late pregnancy, the action of insulin can be 50–70% lower.[295] Also, the production of glucose by the liver can increase 16–30% to meet the needs of the placenta and fetus during pregnancy.[296] The liver has the ability to convert fats and amino acids to glucose to ensure adequate glucose for the developing child. Although the higher blood sugar levels are necessary for the fetus to grow, they also provide a rich source of food for yeast overgrowth, therefore women with chronic yeast overgrowth often experience an increase in the presence and severity of vaginal yeast infections.

Premature labor

Research shows that infections in the womb are a major cause of preterm labor and delivery. The shorter the gestation time before premature labor begins, the greater the likelihood that the expectant mom has an amniotic infection.[297] Bacterial infections were isolated in up to 48% of premature labors[298] and most of these women did not display symptoms of clinical infections. It is important to note that the true percent of pregnant women with silent infections could be much higher due to the fact only a few pathogens were tested. Women who tested positive for amniotic infections were less likely to respond to medications that suppressed premature labor and were more likely to have spontaneous premature rupture of the membranes (PROM).[299]

Certain prostaglandins are known to stimulate abortion and labor and also play an important role in preterm labor.[300] Pregnant women that experienced preterm labor and an infection of the amniotic cavity had higher levels of prostaglandins in the amniotic fluid than women with preterm labor and no infection. These prostaglandins are produced by the expectant mom's tissues in response to the infection but also were produced by the microbes themselves.[301]

Nursing moms

Candida can settle in the breasts and make life really difficult for moms trying to breast feed their babies. Unfortunately, I am speaking from personal experience on this one.

After several months of nursing my third child, I began having issues. One milk duct in one breast would become blocked. It would then become engorged over the next couple of days and finally release. Then a milk duct on the other breast would become blocked, and then engorged and finally release. This fluctuated back and forth from one breast to the other like clockwork. It was very painful and I was so frustrated. I was almost ready to give up breast feeding.

My doctor prescribed a course of antibiotics which didn't help. I visited one naturopath after the next with no relief. One naturopath gave me homeopathic remedies and told me that I was probably suffering from anxiety of some kind. I had successfully nursed two children in the past so I think that I had a pretty good idea of how to breast feed. Now I can chuckle at his response but at the time I couldn't believe what came out of his mouth. Other naturopaths prescribed creams, oral remedies, and light therapy, none of which helped. I was running out of options. Because of my history with yeast overgrowth I suspected that yeast might be the culprit and so in a desperate final attempt I asked my doctor if I could try an antifungal medication rather than antibiotic. He agreed. I took one dose of the antifungal drug Fluconazole, discarded my milk for the recommended amount of time and never experienced this problem again. I continued to nurse my son for another 6 months and stopped nursing when I felt it was the right time.

ABNORMAL FATIGUE?

If you suffer with abnormal fatigue, shortness of breath, headaches, irritability, or dizziness, have your blood iron checked.[302] Iron deficiency anemia is a relatively common blood disorder. Doctors will routinely test hemoglobin levels and red blood cell counts, but often don't test ferritin levels. Ferritin, or stored iron, should also be measured because ferritin levels can become low long before a woman is anemic.

If we live in the land of plenty why is iron deficiency anemia so common? Iron deficiency anemia can be caused by blood loss, poor diet or malabsorption of iron from foods.

Heavy or prolonged menstrual periods or irregular bleeding can be caused by infections.[303] Microbes are able to move from the vagina or cervix into the uterus, fallopian tubes, ovaries, or pelvis.[304] In this book we have explored ample research that shows that silent infections are intimately linked with and are the probable cause of many diseases. Therefore, if you suspect that you have a silent infection it is imperative that you address the infection to prevent further blood loss and future iron deficiency anemia.

Digestive disorders are epidemic in North America and we have explored why this is so. People who suffer with poor digestive health and in particular inflammatory disease have a higher risk of suffering with iron deficiency anemia. Many inflammatory diseases can cause iron deficiency anemia because the tissues in the GI tract become inflamed and bleed. Also these diseases cause poor absorption of iron from food.[305]

Chronic yeast overgrowth may directly cause iron deficient anemia by extracting iron from its host. Candida has iron acquisition proteins on its surface that can extract iron from hemoglobin, transferrin, lactoferrin and ferritin.[306] Several reports have shown that people who suffer with chronic Candida infections are also anemic.[307,308]

One study reported a thirteen year old boy who experienced an onset of oral thrush at the age of 1 month, and then developed an ear infection caused by Candida albicans, followed by recurrent upper respiratory tract infections between the ages of 2–3 years old.[309] Other than an iron deficiency and gluten sensitivity the researchers excluded all other immunodeficiencies.[310] This child is a perfect example of someone who was not immunosuppressed and yet suffered with chronic Candidiasis.

Yet another study reported a 4 year old boy who was admitted to the hospital because of suspected celiac disease. He suffered severe anemia. Celiac was ruled out but the child showed signs of severe Candida esophagitis.[311]

How many others who suffer with anemia also suffer chronic yeast/fungal overgrowth and how often is the anemia directly caused by yeast/fungal overgrowth? More research is needed in this area.

If you suffer with iron deficiency anemia and it is a chronic problem, work with your doctor. Have ferritin levels tested and make sure that you take the iron supplement long enough to restore hemoglobin and ferritin levels. If you feel that you have yeast/fungal overgrowth or another silent infection this must be addressed or you will continue to loose iron directly and indirectly from the infection.

ENDOMETRIOSIS

More than 5 million women in the U.S. suffer with endometriosis.[312] It occurs when tissue that behaves like the cells of the tissue that lines the uterus and womb,[313] grows outside the uterus on other organs and structures such as ovaries, fallopian tubes, in the pelvic cavity, and/or many others parts of the body. The cause of endometriosis is unknown. Women that suffer with endometriosis experience fatigue, very painful menstrual cramps, spotting or bleeding between periods, chronic pain in the lower back and pelvis, pain during and after sex, intestinal pain, and possibly infertility.[314]

It is interesting that women with endometriosis have a significantly higher likelihood of suffering with diarrhea, constipation, bloating,[315] allergies, hypothyroidism, chronic fatigue syndrome, fibromyalgia, autoimmune disease, allergies, and asthma.[316] In addition they also suffer with health problems such as frequent yeast infections, and certain cancers such as ovarian, breast endocrine, kidney, thyroid, brain, and colon cancers, and melanoma and non-Hodgkin's lymphoma[317] ... hmm... sounds like many of the same all-too-common complaints from women who suffer with chronic yeast overgrowth.

One explanation for the pain associated with endometriosis and premenstrual cramps may be the production of the prostaglandins by Candida (or another microbe), or by the body in response to the infection. Prostaglandins are powerful hormone-like chemical messengers that can cause pain, inflammation and contraction of the uterus. See the allergy section of this book for more information on Candida and inflammation (page 177).

OVARIAN CYSTS—OUR BODY'S WAY OF CONTAINING INFECTION?

I believe that cysts are just the body's way of containing an infection. One of my clients had ovarian cysts and visited a medical doctor in Canada who treated her cysts by injecting them with saline or salt water solution. She arrived in his office, had the procedure done and a couple of hours later went out for supper with her husband. She had no unpleasant side effects from this procedure. The cysts decreased to the size of a pea and she has never had a problem with them since.

Dr. Alessandro Antonelli et al[318] showed that 36% of the participants in their study who had a simple salt solution (the same concentration found in the body) injected into thyroid cysts were cured of the cysts. They also found that 77% of subjects who had ethanol injected into thyroid cysts were also cured of the cysts. Other studies found that injection of ethanol into liver and renal cysts was an effective treatment.[319]

I believe that this procedure may offer a safe and effective treatment for cysts and I hope that health care providers will research this further.

For many years Dr. Tullio Simoncini, an Italian oncologist, has been flushing cancer tumors with 5% sodium bicarbonate solution—yes, baking soda—but not the baking soda in your kitchen. This doctor uses pharmaceutical grade sodium bicarbonate (without the aluminum) and has a high success rate. This therapy is ridiculously cost effective and is easy to administer. If you wish to research this further you can find many of his lectures, his book, and many happy patients online. Dr. Simoncini believes that cancer is caused by an infection, in particular, a fungal infection.[320]

Once again we see how simple infections are likely the cause of many disorders and conditions that women suffer with. By ignoring the infection and merely treating symptoms, the infection will continue to grow, moving to different parts of the body and causing further health issues in the years to come.

BIRTH CONTROL: IT'S NOT WORKING FOR US

To put it mildly, I may ruffle a few feathers in this section. Even so, I believe that it is important to take a good hard look at tough issues and give them careful thought and personal reflection for the sake of our wellness and the wellness of our young women.

When did we so wholeheartedly buy into the idea that it is okay for us to be guinea pigs and risk our health for the sake of convenient sex and avoiding pregnancy? Many of us are watching what we eat, exercising and taking supplements, and in the next breath popping a small pill or putting a small patch on our body that has the power to completely override our normal hormonal cycle. How can we not consider that overriding our body's natural hormonal cycle with a synthetic toxic drug may harm our health?

Yes, I know that drug companies have assured us that the newer birth control pills or the patch provide lower doses of synthetic hormones and are therefore much safer than the original versions and no longer cause such a significant increased risk of cancer. Didn't they assure us that the first hormone replacement therapy and the original birth control pill were safe? Haven't we learned our lesson after many *safe* drugs have been introduced into the market and later proven to cause serious health consequences and even occasional death? I am not against the use of pharmaceuticals. They can be very useful in treating crisis situations, but if you don't have to put a toxic drug in your body why would you? All drugs are toxic. All drugs have an LD50 (lethal dose, 50%) rating which indicates the amount of the toxic substance that will kill 50% of the population tested.[321] Hopefully by now most of us realize that governments are not able to protect us from harmful drugs.

Did the newfound sexual freedom that came with birth control really make us happier or have we just been conditioned to believe this by media and pharmaceutical companies? We have been sold on the so-called benefits of contraception, but what are the costs?

There are many agendas in the arena of sex and birth control. Sex is a profitable commodity, and TV programs, movies and music videos seduce us into believing that sex is just a self-gratifying physical act that should be enjoyed whenever the urge arises. The government's concern with this philosophy is the high cost of unwanted pregnancies, supporting single moms, and treating sexually transmitted diseases. Pharmaceutical companies save the day with their response "we have something for that." Drugs and vaccines are available to treat many STDs and contraceptives reduce unwanted pregnancies, and of course we have abortions if all else fails. So everything is taken care of... right? ... or not? Let's consider how women and men are dealing with this.

The media's influence has definitely affected our values. Recent surveys show that more women are not married and are more likely to have sexual relationships and births outside of marriage.[322] Although nearly 11 million U.S. women are on the birth control pill and close to the same number of women have opted for sterilization, half of all pregnancies are unintended.[323] Each year, approximately 750,000 American women between the age of 15–19 become pregnant.[324] In 2006, more than 200,000 abortions were performed on these young women.

In 2008 approximately 1.21 million pregnancies in the U.S. ended in abortion and 17% of these abortions were the result of early abortion medication or the abortion pill.[325] In the U.S., abortions are one of the most common surgical procedures.[326] Adverse reactions to the abortion pill include abdominal pain, uterine cramping, headache, diarrhea, dizziness, fatigue, back pain, uterine hemorrhage, fever, viral infections, vaginitis, hypotension, light-headedness, and loss of consciousness.[327]

According to IMS Health Canada, a company that tracks prescriptions, Canadian pharmacies filled out more than 2 million prescriptions for oral contraceptives in 2009.[328] Pharmaceutical companies assure us and our governments that independent studies conducted on their products show that these newer low-dose birth control pills are safe. Yet in 2009, several Canadians launched a class action lawsuit against a pharmaceutical company that manufactures birth control pills. Dozens of women across Canada have suffered blood clots, pulmonary embolisms, gall bladder removals and other serious medical emergencies. These women claim that their health complications were caused by using this particular birth control pill.

Warnings and precautions listed by the pharmaceutical company that sells this particular birth control pill include:

May cause hyperkalemia in high-risk patients; avoid use in patients predisposed to hyperkalemia (eg, renal insufficiency, hepatic dysfunction, adrenal insufficiency). Monitor K+ levels during first cycle with conditions predisposed to hyperkalemia. Increased risk of myocardial infarction (MI), thromboembolic and thrombotic disease, cerebrovascular diseases, vascular disease, breast cancer, cancer of the reproductive organs, gallbladder disease, and hepatic neoplasia. Increased risk of morbidity and mortality in patients with HTN, hyperlipidemia, obesity, and diabetes mellitus (DM). It may also cause benign hepatic adenomas and hepatocellular carcinoma (rarely reported), retinal thrombosis reported, discontinue use if unexplained partial or complete loss of vision occurs, or onset of proptosis or diplopia, papilledema, or retinal vascular lesions develop. May cause glucose intolerance; monitor prediabetic and diabetic patients. May cause fluid retention and increase BP; monitor closely with HTN and d/c if significant elevation of BP occurs. Discontinue with onset or exacerbation of migraine or development of headache with new pattern which is persistent, recurrent and severe. Breakthrough bleeding and spotting reported; rule out malignancy or pregnancy. Monitor closely with hyperlipidemias. Caution in patient with impaired liver function; discontinue if jaundice develops. Monitor closely with depression and discontinue if depression recurs to serious degree. Contact lens wearers may develop visual changes. Perform annual physical exam. Should not be used to induce withdrawal bleeding as a test for pregnancy or to treat threatened or habitual abortion during pregnancy. Use before menarche is not indicated. May affect certain endocrine, LFTs, and blood components in laboratory tests. Does not protect against HIV infection (AIDS) and other STDs.[329]

Why would any woman take this drug? This list of precautions is frightening! It's ironic that we are assured that these drugs are safe, yet the warning and precautions suggest otherwise. How many women actually read up on these drugs before they fill their prescription? Your health is your responsibility. You cannot afford to leave it in the hands of any expert!

Although oral contraceptives are widely used in preventing pregnancy, there is a growing concern among women about their side effects.[330] The Canadian Cancer Society and American Cancer Society both state on their websites that taking the birth control pill increases a woman's risk of breast cancer. Furthermore, the use of oral contraceptives can increase a woman's susceptibility to sexually transmitted diseases and certain genital tract infections.[331] It is interesting that in order for scientists to establish certain infections in lab animals, these animals must be treated with female sex hormones.[332]

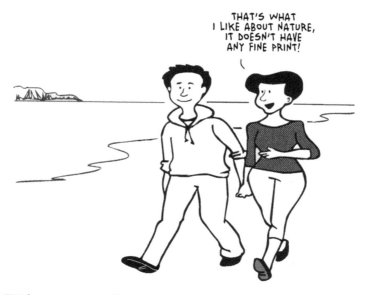

With over 10 million American women and 2 million Canadian women excreting synthetic hormones from oral contraceptives and hormone replacement therapy into our water supply, we must also consider how these hormones affect our environment. As mentioned in the section Minimize Your Toxin Load (page 165), scientists are finding gender confusion in our fish which they believe is the result of synthetic estrogens and xenoestrogens in waste water. Although oral contraceptives may not be the leading source of estrogen pollution in our water supply, their concentration in surface water does pose a health risk to local wildlife.[333] These researchers recommend that efforts should be made to reduce the sources of all estrogenic substances in our water supply.

About 5% of women that take the birth control pill become pregnant.[334] Birth control pills work by "preventing ovulation, and producing changes in cervical mucus (increasing difficulty of sperm entry into the uterus) and endometrium (reducing the likelihood of implantation).[335] There is a heated debate among scientists as to how often conception takes place while a woman is on the birth control pill and how often the pill prevents implantation. If this is the case, then the birth control pill acts not only as a contraceptive but occasionally as an agent that causes abortion.

About 23% of all pregnancies end in abortion and nearly half of abortions occur in women in their twenties. Proponents for abortion claim that there is no evidence that abortions cause mental disorders in women, but research is showing something very different. Natalie P. Mota et al[336] found a strong relationship between abortions and mental disorders. Clinical implications from this study include:

1. Some women with a history of abortion develop emotional problems, and clinicians should assess for mental disorders, particularly substance use disorders (SUDs) in these women.

2. Clinicians should screen for a history of abortion in women presenting with mood, anxiety, or SUDs as a potential contributing factor.

3. Women presenting for abortion should be screened for a history of violence.

Dr. Priscilla K. Coleman[337] has compiled a list of over 30 current scientific studies showing an abortion-mental health connection. These peer-reviewed studies show a relationship between abortions and mood, anxiety, depression, substance use disorders, post-traumatic stress, subsequent relationship difficulties, physiological stress in men and women, sleeping disorders and an increased risk of suicide.

If the birth control pill and abortion are detrimental to a woman's health, what are our options? I believe that if our goal is complete wellness, then maybe we should try another approach.

Food for thought

My intention is not to suggest what any woman should do, but to challenge women to evaluate their behaviors and determine if these behaviors promote wellness in their life. Wellness involves much more than just our physical state. It includes our emotional, psychological, physical, and spiritual well-being.

Is it possible that many women and men bought into a notion of sex that wasn't true? Maybe this new attitude of sexual freedom and self-gratification was good for the media industry's profits, but not necessarily good for us. Is it possible that we thought this was what we wanted but now have come to realize that moving in and out of sexually intimate relationships is very painful because sex is more than a physical act? It is an emotional and spiritual connection. Women are nurturers by design. We give life and the price we pay for unwanted pregnancies and abortion is far too great to bear.

What if we choose to reserve that emotional and spiritual connection for someone who loves us enough, and we love them enough to publicly and legally commit to each other for life, before we make that spiritual connection? What if we make the decision to practice abstinence and preserve sex for that special person who has committed to us for life publicly and legally?

The U.S. government Women's Health site reports that abstinence "is the only sure way to prevent pregnancy and protect against sexually transmitted infections (STIs), including HIV."[338] Abstinence protects us from the deep level of emotional pain from broken relationships. It is hard enough when a relationship ends, but adding the spiritual connection of sex takes the pain of the breakup to a much higher level.

Can we adhere to abstinence on our own? Possibly. But I believe that with God in the picture our success will be much greater. This might all seem idealistic, but I believe that this approach offers the greatest reward and emotional success with respect to relationships and pregnancy.

For those who want to explore a healthy alternative to contraception, you should research the Creighton model.[339] Fehring, Lawrence and Philpot stated that this method is effective when used to avoid pregnancy.[340] We have used this method successfully in our marriage and found that it is very effective in avoiding pregnancy; and when the time was right to conceive, it was easy to determine the time of ovulation and become pregnant. In order for this method to be effective you and your partner must be instructed by qualified teachers. If the couple decides to have intercourse during the woman's time of fertility, they are using the method to achieve pregnancy.

TREAT YOUR PARTNER, TOO

If you have suffered for years with symptoms of chronic yeast over-growth and you have been in the same long-term committed relationship, chances are your partner also has yeast overgrowth. You and your partner are probably dealing with different degrees of yeast overgrowth and in different parts of the body. It is really important to treat both parties involved in an intimate relationship in order to experience long term success.

Become a Wellness Champion

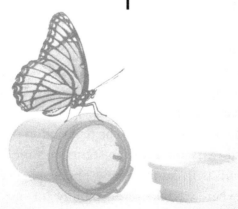

IN REVIEW

We have covered a lot of ground. We have taken a hard, honest look at where our health is at, how we got here, what is stopping us from moving forward. Also, we have explored what our present approach to health care is costing us both financially and with respect to our quality of life. We have also discussed a solution that works—building the Four Pillars of Wellness:

- Pillar #1 Optimize Nutrition
- Pillar #2 Minimize Silent Infections
- Pillar #3 Minimize Your Toxin Load
- Pillar #4 Build a Healthy Lifestyle

Governments have sounded the alarm that our health care systems are in a state of crisis. As disease trends and pharmaceutical and medical costs continue to rise, and as more baby boomers reach retirement, health care costs will continue to rise at an unsustainable rate. In Canada this will likely translate into higher taxes, longer wait times and fewer services covered. In the U.S., health care costs could become the new mortgage payment.

Many of us are dissatisfied with our quality of life and are searching for ways to improve it. We realize that living with chronic illness is horrible and that there must be a better way.

We have one of two options. The first option is to stick our heads in the sand and carry on with the status quo until we hit the brick wall. The second is to adopt a new philosophy; one of prevention and wellness, where we take responsibility for our health and work to minimize our dependence on an unsustainable health care system. Sickness is expensive and we will have to pay for it one way or another unless enough of us change our direction, take responsibility for our health and become Wellness Champions. That meaningful change will come is inevitable, but what will *you* choose?

If your choice is prevention and wellness, then focus on building your Four Pillars of Wellness and adopt the mindset of a Wellness

Champion (as described on page 24 & 219). Just as a table needs four solid legs, the Four Pillars of Wellness are equally important for optimal health. Wellness requires a holistic approach. There is no quick fix. If one pillar is not solid, the wellness you experience will be limited.

Nutrition is the foundation for wellness. We must first support the body by providing it with necessary and essential nutrients from whole foods and supplements created from *real food* so that it can do what it is designed to do, which is build, restore, and defend.

Dysbiosis awareness has been a key missing piece of the wellness puzzle. If dysbiosis is not dealt with and our natural defenses aren't restored, success will be limited. I believe this has been a major stumbling block for many people.

Although the term dysbiosis may be new to many of us, dysbiosis is epidemic. It has been shown that the prevalence of dysbiosis is largely initiated by the overuse of antibiotics and certain other pharmaceuticals, and then fueled by our diets rich in processed carbohydrates.

> To support the body naturally so that it can do what it is designed to do —what a simple concept!

There is sufficient evidence to show that yeast overgrowth causes disease in people who were not originally immune suppressed, and that yeast/fungal overgrowth directly suppresses our immune system. Over time as the infection becomes pervasive, the immune system will become increasingly suppressed.

Because the medical community believes that yeast overgrowth is not a concern for the vast majority of people, it was important to provide scientific evidence showing that yeast overgrowth is a true concern and that yeast overgrowth can clearly make us sick. My hope is that you will share this information with your health care professional in a respectful and tactful manner. Although this book has focused on yeast and fungi, dysbiosis often involves other parasites. Working with an experienced health care professional will help you determine if other parasites are involved and which treatment(s) will

BECOME A WELLNESS CHAMPION

be most effective.

It is really quite simple: from the moment we are born until the moment we die, the world of microbes is trying to take us out. Our game plan:

1. Protect and constantly restore our natural defenses (including the good guys)
2. Keep the population of the bad guys in our bodies to a minimum
3. Maintain a strong immune system

All three steps of this game plan can be accomplished by building four solid pillars of wellness. For the most part, the longer we keep the bad guys at bay, the longer we will live and the better our quality of life will be. I believe it's that simple.

We will soon witness an explosion in probiotic research and many new products will emerge in the marketplace. Probiotics may offer the biggest hope for restoring balance in the GI tract, but be aware that these supplements will receive their share of marketing hype. The consumer will find probiotics added to many different foods but the therapeutic value will be minimal of any. In order to benefit from taking probiotics you must take an adequate dose of the right strains of safe bacteria or other microbes. Work with an experienced health care professional to get the best results.

> From the moment we are born until the moment we die, the world of microbes is trying to take us out.

Wellness requires a proactive approach where we support the body to operate at its peak, not search for a quick fix to mask a problem. The body is highly complex and intelligently designed, and science has much to learn about how it functions.

YOU COULD BE YOUR OWN WORST ENEMY!

You must get out of your own way! Erroneous beliefs are the biggest threat to your success. Take an honest look at your beliefs around wellness. Do they serve you or are they keeping you stuck? The level of wellness that you experience at this time is the product of your beliefs. Your beliefs are literally making your decisions for you.

Discuss your beliefs around wellness with a health care professional, coach or mentor that you trust and whom you feel is really succeeding in the area of wellness. They will help you determine if you have beliefs that are holding you back.

What is your wellness goal and how strong is your intention? Your goal must be crystal clear and your intention incredibly strong. The strength of your intention will come from

> We must determine what is interfering with our body's ability to run optimally and address this.

an unyielding *why*. Why must you accomplish your goal? What are the benefits if you accomplish your goal? And what are the costs if you fail? The more emotions you employ the stronger your why will be. A coach or mentor can also help you build a strong intention so that you will succeed. Please don't skip this. Your beliefs will either support or obstruct your success.

BECOME A WELLNESS CHAMPION!

As a Wellness Champion you have made the decision to take responsibility for your health and become proactive. Adopting a healthy lifestyle is the only option for you. You understand that wellness is earned by following basic fundamental principles—The Four Pillars of Wellness. You choose to minimize your dependence on an unsustainable health care system. Quality of life is very important to you, and optimal health will allow you to do the things you love to do. An active life is important to you but balance is something that you are constantly aware of and strive for. You are purpose-driven and share this message of hope with others who are searching for answers. You are a true champion!

IT DOESN'T MATTER WHERE YOU START... JUST START!

It doesn't matter if you related to the Delusionally Healthy, Not-so-relieved Diagnosed, or Hypochondriac health club. You can begin to change your destiny by making the decision to become a Wellness Champion today! I have worked with a diverse group of people with diverse challenges. It doesn't matter if your challenges are great or small. Just start! Becoming a Wellness Champion is a journey. Take consistent simple steps and don't beat yourself up if you slip along the way. As long as you are moving forward, you are succeeding. Celebrate your success!

WE DRIVE THE WELLNESS MARKET

As more of us become Wellness Champions and choose a holistic approach to health, our health care system and food industry will change to meet our needs. As we search out and choose higher quality produce and whole foods, producers and growers will follow our lead. We are already witnessing the start of this as many grocery stores are expanding their certified organic selection and offer customers healthy choice sections in their stores. As more of us make healthier choices, we will continue to see an ever-expanding selection of healthy choices available to us.

As a Wellness Champion, you will wake up to a new world of possibilities. You will feel and look younger and take on a healthy glow. In your renewed state, you will see your world through a new set of eyes and will feel inspired! You will live your life instead of letting life run you. You will be in the game rather than merely a spectator. Your energy and stamina will soar and you will be energized to take up hobbies that you have always wanted to do, enjoy time and activities with your family or friends or maybe even take on an extreme sport. You will find that you live with passion and purpose.

As your family, friends and co-workers see the change in you, they will be inspired by you and curious to know what you are doing. This will give you the opportunity to impact their lives. If you are a parent, you have the amazing opportunity to pass this knowledge onto your children and equip them to enjoy wellness throughout their life. This is your opportunity to leave a legacy. If being a Wellness Champion changes your life and the life of just one other person... isn't that alone worth it?

MEET REAL LIFE WELLNESS CHAMPIONS

The following are examples of people who are true Wellness Champions. As you read their stories, you may be tempted to ask, "What is the secret to their success? What were the one or two things they did to achieve their success?" The fact is, it's impossible to answer that question. Each person is unique. Each person has a unique genetic make-up and has been exposed to a different environment. Also, each person holds a unique set of beliefs and values. For years these individuals have demonstrated their commitment to being Wellness Champions by continually reinforcing their Four Pillars of Wellness. Life continues to bring new challenges, but their dedication to being a Wellness Champion allows them to live a high quality life in spite of the new challenges. In being a Wellness Champion we never arrive or reach the top. Being a Wellness Champion requires that we take on a new attitude, one of personal responsibility for our wellness, and we become more aware of what promotes or hinders our wellness.

Chris

Chris suffered with debilitating pain from fibromyalgia and wanted to lose some weight. As she took charge of her wellness and began building her Four Pillars of Wellness, her world transformed. She is now at her ideal body weight, and looks 10 years younger. She didn't diet. Her focus is wellness. Chris is no longer disabled with pain and radiates a healthy glow. Her friends are so inspired by her transformation that many have started to adopt healthier lifestyles. They want what she has. Wellness is contagious!

Ryan

I have known Ryan for several years. He is an amazing 39 year old Kelowna triathlete. Just as there are extreme athletes, Ryan is an extreme Wellness Champion. His dedication to wellness is not the result of poor health, but because of his passion for peak performance. He has already completed the Penticton Ironman Canada Triathlon 5 times. This triathlon includes a 2.4 mile swim, a 112 mile bike ride and a 26.2 mile run.

Ryan's master plan for 2012 is to set a record climbing Mount Everest without oxygen and climbing all seven summits not once, but twice.[341] In order to perform at such a high level, Ryan is considerably more disciplined with respect to wellness than the vast majority of people his age.

This year Ryan will continue to prepare for the Mount Everest adventure by first completing the Boise Marathon in May, then climbing Mount Whitney in California (the highest mountain in the contiguous U.S.), later climbing the peaks in Colorado in September, then doing a practice run to the base camp in Nepal in October, and finally climbing Cerro Aconcagua in the South American Andes twice—in November and December.[342] Ryan shows us that Wellness Champions are motived by very different passions. He is a genuine role model in the areas of leadership, active living and wellness. He also loves to encourage others to reach for excellence.

Barb

Barb is one of the most positive people I have ever met. I met Barb about 7 years ago. At that time she was really struggling with multiple sclerosis; it had affected her cognition and her ability to walk. I watched Barb's health transform over the next few months. Her quality of life and brain function improved so much that she returned to her passions, including teaching Trec (a unique equestrian sport), and trail riding with her horses and mules. She is once again able to do what she loves to do. Barb inspires everyone she meets.

Carey

Carey is an amazing example of a Wellness Champion. Carey had a history of colitis which progressed into Crohn's years ago. With a lot of work on her part, Carey has been able to keep the Crohn's in remission for the past 12 years without the use of pharmaceuticals or surgery. She has also been in two serious car accidents, neither of which were her fault, but the most recent accident almost took her life. Many of us would have just given up, but her drive and commitment to wellness is truly an inspiration. Carey uses an integrative approach to wellness. One of her health care providers told Carey that she was his sickest patient at the start of the year (because of an automotive accident), but had improved the most by the end of the year. Carey's passion for life and love for her son drove her to seek out therapies and supplements that would complement the care of her doctor and give her back the quality of life she wanted. She radiates health, lives an active life and enjoys the outdoors. She has touched the lives of literally thousands of people and is a true inspiration.

WE ALL DESERVE IT

Become a Wellness Champion and share your story. Inspire others who are searching for hope. Others need to hear your story.

It would seem that my diagnosis of MS would have been the worst event of my life, and at that time it was. I was filled with sheer hopelessness and fear. It felt that I no longer had a future and that I was destined to be a burden to my family. Although there were many trying times at the start of this journey, this event changed the course of my life. The small amount of knowledge that I have gained has created up an opportunity for me to significantly impact the lives of hundreds of others and my goal is to reach many more. I truly don't have all the answers, but what I have learned over the past 20+ years has profoundly improved my quality of life and has the potential to benefit everyone.

My faith in God really carried me through that time. I thank God for showing me a world of possibilities that I didn't know existed. I did take action and the result has not only benefited me but also my family, friends and the clients I coach.

But what will it take to get you to realize that you will miss out on so much in your life unless you choose to become a Wellness Champion? You deserve a vibrant full life, but that might not be enough to motivate some of you at this time. Your family deserves it and our environment and society in general deserve your commitment to take responsibility for your health. Perhaps you're motivated by the opportunity to buck the system that has so clearly not been driven by the goal of promoting wellness.

My hope is that the information in this book has inspired and motivated you to become a Wellness Champion, whatever your reasons. We all deserve optimal health.

I invite you to join me on this journey of building the Four Pillars of Wellness and becoming a Wellness Champion. Subscribe to my video blog at www.becomeawellnesschampion.com, where I will share wellness nuggets. Join our Facebook group *Become a Wellness Champion* and share your success with others. Let's change the world together, one person at a time!

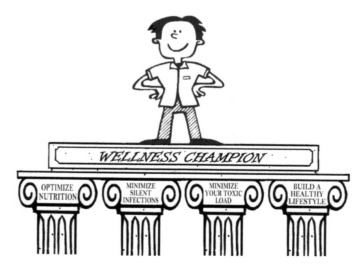

REFERENCES

SECTION ONE

1 Organization for Economic Co-operation and Development (OECD). (2010). *Growing health spending puts pressure on government budgets, according to OECD Health Data 2010.* Retrieved from: http://www.oecd.org/document/11/0,3746,en_21571361_ 44315115_45549771_1_1_1_1,00.html

2 Ibid.

3 IBM. (2006). *Healthcare 2015: Win-win or lose-lose? IBM Global Business Services Healthcare—A portrait and a path to successful transformation.* Retrieved from http:// www-935.ibm.com/services/us/gbs/bus/pdf/healthcare2015-win-win_or_lose-lose.pdf

4 DiMasi, J.A., Hansen, R.W., & Grabowski, H.G. (2003). The price of innovation: new estimates of drug development costs. *Journal of Health Economics*, 22(2), 151–185.

5 Organization for Economic Co-operation and Development (OECD). (2010). *Growing health spending puts pressure on government budgets, according to OECD Health Data 2010.* Retrieved from: http://www.oecd.org/ document/11/0,3746,en_21571361_ 44315115_45549771_1_1_1_1,00.Html

6 Skinner, B., & Rovere, M. (2007). *An unsustainable system. Why are we paying more and getting less?* Fraser Institute. Fraser Forum. Retrieved from http://www.fraserinstitute.org/ uploadedFiles/fraser-ca/Content/research-news/research/articles/an-unsustainable-system.pdf

7 IBM. (2006). *Healthcare 2015: Win-win or lose-lose? IBM Global Business Services Healthcare—A portrait and a path to successful transformation.* Retrieved from http:// www-935.ibm.com/services/us/gbs/bus/pdf/healthcare2015-win-win_or_lose-lose.pdf

8 Stuart, N., & Adams, J. (2007). The sustainability of Canada's healthcare system: A framework for advancing the debate. Longwoods Review, *Healthcare Quarterly*, 10(2), 96–103. Retrieved from http://www.longwoods.com/content/18839

9 Organization for Economic Co-operation and Development (OECD). (2010). *Growing health spending puts pressure on government budgets, according to OECD Health Data 2010.* Retrieved from: http://www.oecd.org/document/11/0,3746,en_21571361_ 44315115_45549771_1_1_1_1,00.html

10 World Health Organization. (2000). *The World Health Report 2000: health systems: improving performance.* Retrieved from http://www.who.int/whr/2000/en/

Organization for Economic Co-operation and Development. (2006). *OECD health data 2006: Statistics and indicators for 30 countries.* (15th edition). Paris: OECD Publishing.

11 IBM. (2006). *Healthcare 2015: Win-win or lose-lose? IBM Global Business Services Healthcare—A portrait and a path to successful transformation.* Retrieved from http:// www-935.ibm.com/services/us/gbs/bus/pdf/healthcare2015-win-win_or_lose-lose.pdf

12 Organization for Economic Co-operation and Development (OECD). (2005). *OECD countries spend only 3% of healthcare budgets on prevention, public awareness.* Retrieved from http://www.oecd.org/document/0/0,2340,en_2649_201185_35625856 _1_1_1_1,00.html

13 B.C. Ministry of Health. Ministry of Health Services. (2011). *MSP*. Retrieved from http://www.health.gov.bc.ca/msp/infoben/premium.html

14 Government of Alberta Health and Wellness. (2010). *Plan benefits and services*. Retrieved from http://www.health.alberta.ca/AHCIP/plan-benefits.html

15 Ontario Ministry of Revenue. (2010). *Ontario health premium rate chart*. Retrieved from http://www.rev.gov.on.ca/en/tax/healthpremium/rates.html

16 Canadian Institute of Health. (2008). *The cost of acute care hospital stays by medical condition in Canada 2004–2005*. Retrieved from http://secure.cihi.ca/cihiweb/products/nhex_acutecare07_e.pdf

17 B.C. Ministry of Health. (2010). *MSP. General practice*. Retrieved from http://www.health.gov.bc.ca/msp/infoprac/physbilling/payschedule/pdf/7.%20general_practice.pdf

18 U.S. Department of Health and Human Services, Agency for Healthcare Research and Quality (AHRQ). (2007). *Primary care doctors account for nearly half of physician visits but less than one–third of expenses*. Retrieved from http://www.ahrq.gov/news/nn/nn042507.htm

19 Sierles, F.S., Brodkey, A.C., Cleary, L.M., McCurdy, F.A., Mintz, M., Frank, J., Lynn, D.J., Chao, J., Morgenstern, B.Z., Shore, W., Woodard, J.L. (2005). Medical students exposure to and attitudes about drug company interactions: a national survey. *Journal of the Medical Association*, 294, 1034–1042.

20 Sufrin, C.B., & Ross, J.S. (2008). Pharmaceutical industry marketing: Understanding its impact on women's health. *Obstetrical & Gynecological Survey*, 63(9), 585–596.

21 York University. (2008). *Big Pharma spends more on advertising than research and development, study finds*. Science Daily. Retrieved from http://www.sciencedaily.com/releases/2008/01/080105140107.htm

22 Barfett, J., Lanting, B., Lee, J., Lee, M., Ng, V., & Simkhovitch, P. (2004). Pharmaceutical marketing to medical students: the student perspective. *McGill Journal of Medicine*, 8, 21–27.

23 Sibbald, B. (2001). Doctors asked to take pledge to shun drug company freebies. *Canadian Medical Association Journal*, 164(4), 531.

24 Barfett, J., Lanting, B., Lee, J., Lee, M., Ng, V., & Simkhovitch, P. (2004). Pharmaceutical marketing to medical students: the student perspective. *McGill Journal of Medicine*, 8, 21–27.

25 Lexchin, J. (2008). *CME and the pharmaceutical industry: do those who have the gold make the rules?* School of Health Policy & Management, York University. Emergency Department, University Health Network. Retrieved from http://www.caep.ca/caep2010/presentations/Tuesday-1045-Controversy-Lexchin_Joel.pdf

26 Ibid.

27 Kondro, W. (2008). Industry handouts: enough is enough. *Canadian Medical Association Journal*, 178(13), 1651–1652.

28 Morgan, S., Black, C., Barer, M., Reid, R., Evans, R., & Agnew, J. (2004). *Drug expenditures in Canada: a population-based analysis of trends and causes*. AcademyHealth. Retrieved from http://gateway.nlm.nih.gov/MeetingAbstracts/ma?f=103624457.html

29 Lundy, J. (2010). *Prescription drug costs*. Fraiser Family Foundation. Retrieved from http://www.kff.org/rxdrugs/upload/3057-08.pdf

30 Organization for Economic Co-operation and Development (OECD). (2005). *Health care at a glance. OECD indicators 2005*. Retrieved from http://www.oecd.org/dataoecd/58/47/35624825.pdf

31 Canadian Institute of Health. (2010). *Drug expenditure in Canada 1985–2009.* Retrieved from http://secure.cihi.ca/cihiweb/products/dex_1985_to_2009_e.pdf

32 World Health Organization. (1997). *Health performance rank by country.* Retrieved from http://www.photius.com/rankings/world_health_performance_ranks.html

33 Kimbuende, E., Ranji, U., & Salganicoff, A. (2010). *Prescription drug costs.* Fraiser Family Foundation. Retrieved from: http://www.kaiseredu.org/topics_im.aspid=352& parentID=68&imID=1#_edn2b

34 York University. (2008). *Big Pharma spends more on advertising than research and development, study finds.* Science Daily. Retrieved from http://www.sciencedaily.com/ releases/2008/01/080105140107.htm

35 Ibid.

36 Avorn, J. (2007). Paying for drug approvals—Who is using whom? *New England Journal of Medicine, 356*(17), 1697–1700.

37 Ibid.

38 Permacology Productions Pty Ltd. (2010). *Food matters. You are what you eat.* [DVD]. Available from http://www.foodmatters.tv/_webapp/The%20Film

39 Favaro, A., St. Philip, E. (2007). *Small molecule offers hope for cancer treatment.* CTV News. Retrieved from http://www.ctv.ca/CTVNews/CTVNewsAt11/20070116/cancer_dca_070116/

40 University of Alberta. Faculty of Medicine and Dentistry. The University of Alberta Discovery. The Official University of Alberta DCA Website. (2007). *DCA research information.* Received from http://www.dca.med.ualberta.ca/Home/ Updates/2007-03-15_Update.cfm

41 Chen, Q., Espey, M.J., Sun, A.Y., Pooput, C., Kirk, K.L., Krishna, M.C., Khosh, D.B., Drisko, J., & Levine, M. (2008). Pharmacologic doses of ascorbate act as a prooxidant and decrease growth of aggressive tumor xenografts in mice. *Proceedings of the National Academy of Sciences, 105*(32), 11105–11109.

42 Padayatty, S.J., Riordan, H.D., Hewitt, S.M., Katz, A., Hoffer, L.J., & Levine, M. (2006). Intravenously administered vitamin C as cancer therapy: three cases. *Canadian Medical Association Journal, 174*(7), 937–947.

43 World Health Organization website. (2010). *Health topics. Fact sheet. Diabetes.* Retrieved from http://www.who.int/mediacentre/factsheets/fs312/en/

44 American Heart Association website. (2010). *Cardiovascular disease statistics.* Retrieved from http://www.americanheart.org/presenter.jhtml?identifier=4478

45 Canadian Cancer Society website. (2010). *General cancer statistics for 2010.* Received from http://www.cancer.ca/Canada- wide/About%20cancer/Cancer%20 statistics/ Stats%20at%20a%20glance/General%20cancer%20 stats.aspx?sc_lang=en

46 Kogan, M.D., Blumberg, S.J., Schieve, L.A., Boyle, C.A., Perrin, J.M., Ghandour, R.M., Singh, G.K., Strickland, B.B., Trevathan, E., & Van Dyck, P.C. (2009). Prevalence of parent-reported diagnosis of autism spectrum disorder among children in the US, 2007. *Pediatrics, 124*(5), 1395–1403. doi:10.1542/peds.2009–1522

47 National Institute of Health. (2009). *Summary of research activties by disease category. Autoimmune diseases.* Retrieved from http://report.nih.gov/biennialreport/PDF/ Ch2_Autoimmune.pdf

48 US Department of Health and Human Services. Office on Women's Health. (2010). *Autoimmune diseases overview.* Retrieved from http://www.womenshealth.gov/faq/ autoimmune-diseases.pdf

49 Ibid.

50 Ibid.

51 Nakazawa, D. (2008).*The Autoimmune Epidemic*. New York: Simon & Schuster.

52 Ibid.

53 Merck. The Merck Manuals Online Medical Library. (2008). *Antibiotics*. Retrieved from http://www.merckmanuals.com/home/sec17/ch192/ ch192a. html?qt=antibiotics&alt=sh#sec17-ch192-ch192a-422

54 Margolis, D.J., Fanelli, M., Hoffstad, O., & Lewis, J.D. (2010). Potential association between the oral tetracycline class of antimicrobials used to treat acne and inflammatory bowel disease. *American Journal Gastroenterology*, 105(12), 2610–2616. doi:10.1038/ ajg.2010.303

55 Margolis, D.J., Bowe, W.P., Hoffstad, O., & Berlin, J.A. (2005). Antibiotic treatment of acne may be associated with upper respiratory tract infections. *Archives of Dermatology*, 141, 1132–1136.

56 Card, T., Logan, R.F.A., Rodrigues, L.C., & Wheeler, J.G. (2004). Antibiotic use and the development of Crohn's disease. *Gut*, 53, 246–250. doi:10.1136/gut.2003.025239

57 American College of Gastroenterology. (2011). *Common GI problems: Volume 1*. Retrieved from http://www.acg.gi.org/patients/cgp/cgpvol1.asp

58 Canadian Digestive Health Foundation. (2009). *Establishing digestive health as a priority for Canadians. National digestive disorders prevalence & impact study report*. Retrieved from http://www.cdhf.ca/pdfs/CDHF_National_Prevalence_Impact_Study_ Report_Nov_2009.pdf

59 Velicer, C.M., Heckbert, S.R., Lampe, J.W., Potter, J.D., Robertson, C.A., & Taplin, S.H. (2004). Antibiotic use in relation to the risk of breast cancer. *Journal of the American Medical Association*, 291(7), 827–835.

60 Merck. The Merck Manuals Online Medical Library. (2008). *Antibiotics*. Retrieved from http://www.merckmanuals.com/home/sec17/ch192/ ch192a.html?qt=antibiotics &alt=sh#sec17-ch192-ch192a-422

61 Webb, N. (2003). *The cost of being sick*. Orem, Utah: Sound Concepts Inc.

62 Heart and Stroke Foundation. (2010). *A perfect storm of heart disease looming on our horizon*. Retrieved from http://www.heartandstroke.com/atf/cf/%7B99452D8B-E7F1- 4BD6-A57D- B136CE6C95BF%7D/Jan23_EN_ReportCard.pdf

63 Heart and Stroke Foundation. (2010). *What is killing our kids?* Retrieved from http://www.heartandstroke.on.ca/atf/cf/%7B33C6FA68-B56B-4760-ABC6- D85B2D02EE71%7D/AR_09_Final_web_2.pdf?src=link

64 Klepper, B., & Kibble, D.C. (2010). *If employers walk away from health coverage*. Kaiser Health News. Henry J. Kaiser Family Foundation. Retrieved from http://www. kaiserhealthnews.org/Columns/2010/November/112410klepperkibbe.aspx

65 Rovner, J. (2010). *Caution: High deductible plans might be bad for your health*. Kaiser Health News. Henry J. Kaiser Family Foundation. Retrieved from http://www.kaiser healthnews.org/Stories/2010/November/24/health-insurance-high-deductible- npr. aspx?utm_source=feedburner&utm_ medium=feed&utm_campaign=Feed%3A+New- From KaiserHealthNews+%28New+From+Kaiser+Health+News%29

66 Webb, N. (2003). *The cost of being sick*. Orem, Utah: Sound Concepts Inc.

67 Ibid.

Section Two

68 Chang, A.C., & Page, A.L. (2000). Trace elements slowly accumulating, depleting in soils. *California Agriculture, 54*(2), 49–55. doi: 10.3733/ca.v054n02p49

69 Ibid.

70 Thomas, D. (2007). The mineral depletion of foods available to us as a nation (1940 – 2002). A review of the 6th edition of McCance and Widdowson, *Nutrition & Health*, 19, 21–55.

71 Ibid.

72 Schaffer, M. (2001). *Waste lands: The threat of toxic fertilizer.* Toxics Policy Advocate. Retrieved from http://www.pirg.org/toxics/reports/wastelands/

73 Ibid.

74 Chang, A.C., & Page, A.L. (2000). Trace elements slowly accumulating, depleting in soils. *California Agriculture, 54*(2), 49–55. doi: 10.3733/ca.v054n02p49

75 Davis, D.R. (2009). Declining fruit and vegetable nutrient composition: What is the evidence? *HortScience, 44*(1), 15–19.

76 Davis, R.D., Epp, M.D., & Riordan, H.D. (2004). Changes in USDA food composition data for 43 garden crops, 1950 to 1999. *Journal of the American College of Nutrition*, 23(6), 669–682.

77 Goldman, I.L., Kader, A.A., & Heintz, M.S. (1999). Influence of production, handling, and storage on phytonutrient content of foods. *Nutritional Reviews, 57*(9), 46–52. doi: 10.1111/j.1753–4887.1999.tb01807.x

78 Wold, A., Rosenfeld, H., Holte, K., Baugerød, H., Blomhoff, R., & Haffner, K. (2004). Colour of post-harvest ripened and vine ripened tomatoes (Lycopersicon esculentum Mill.) as related to total antioxidant capacity and chemical composition. *International Journal of Food Science & Technology, 39*(3), 295–302. doi:10.1111/j.1365–2621.2004.00784.x.

79 O'Connor, A. (2009). *Refrigeration preserves the nutrients of fruits and vegetables.* New York Times. Retrieved from http://query.nytimes.com/gst/fullpage.html?res=9800E1D8123CF93BA15754C0A96F9C8B63

80 Christian, J. (2002). *Charts: nutrients changes in vegetables and fruits, 1951 to 1999.* CTV News. Retrieved from http://www.ctv.ca/CTVNews/Health/20020705/favaro_nutrients_chart_020705/

81 Ibid.

82 Mayer, A.M. (1997). Historical changes in the mineral content of fruits and vegetables. *British Food Journal, 99*(6), 207–211.

83 Davis, D.R. (2009). Declining fruit and vegetable nutrient composition: What is the evidence? *HortScience, 44*(1), 15–19.

84 US Department of Agriculture (USDA). (2005). *Dietary guidelines for Americans 2005.* Retrieved from http://www.health.gov/dietaryguidelines/dga2005/document/pdf/DGA2005.pdf

85 Proevity Continuing Education Group. (2009). *How to evaluate vitamin and mineral products. What healthcare professionals want to know.* Retrieved from www.proevity cme.com

86 United Sates Department of Agriculture. National Agricultural Library. (2011). *What is organic production?* Retrieved from http://www.nal.usda.gov/afsic/pubs/ofp/ofp.shtml

87 Environmental Working Group. (2010). *EWG's shopper's guide to pesticides.* Retrieved from http://www.foodnews.org/

88 Ibid.

89 Environmental Working Group. (2010). *EWG's shopper's guide to pesticides.* Retrieved from http://www.foodnews.org/

90 Linus Pauling Intitute. Micronutrient Information Center. (2010). *Phytosterols.* Retrieved from http://lpi.oregonstate.edu/infocenter/phytochemicals.html

91 Cabezas, A. (1994). The origins of glycobiology. *Biochemical Education,* 22(1), 3–7.

92 Murray, R.K., Granner, D.K., Mayes, P.A., Rodwell, V.W. (2003). Glycoprotiens. In Foltin, J., Ransom, J., Oransky, J.M. (26th Ed) *Harper's Illustrated Biochemistry,* (pp. 514–534). United States of America: McGraw-Hill Companies Inc.

93 MedicineNet. (2011). *Definition of glycoprotein.* Retrieved from http://www.med terms.com/script/main/art.asp?articlekey=16842

94 Cohen, J. (2003). Glycomics. *MIT's Magazine of Innovation Technology Review,* 106(1), 46–48.

95 Best, T., Kemps, E., & Bryan, J. (2010). Saccharide effects on cognition and well-being in middle-aged adults: a randomized controlled trial. *Developmental Neuropsychology,* 35(1), 66–80.

96 Stancil, A.N., & Hicks, L.H. (2009). Glyconutrients and perception, cognition, and memory. *Perceptual and Motor Skills,* 10, 259–270.

97 Wang, C., Szabo, J.S., & Dykman, R.A. (2004). Effects of a carbohydrate supplement upon resting brain activity. *Integrative Physiological and Behavioral Science,* 39, 126–138.

98 Wang, C., Pivik, R.T., & Dykman, R.A. (2002). *Effects of a glyconutritional supplement on brain potentials associated with language processing.* Federation Proceedings: Experimental Biology Meeting, New Orleans, Louisiana.

99 Rollins, J. (2010). *Glyconutrients: the most controversial discovery in modern health care.* The Atlanta Voice Newspaper. Special Addition.

100 Ibid.

101 Proevity Continuing Education Group. (2009). *How to evaluate vitamin and mineral products. What healthcare professionals want to know.* Retrieved from www.proevity cme.com

102 Dickinson, A., Boyon, N., & Shao, A. (2009). Physicians and nurses use and recommend dietary supplements: report of a survey. *Nutrition Journal Research,* 8(29), 1–8. Retrieved from http://www.nutritionj.com/content/pdf/1475-2891-8-29.pdf

103 Goodman, G.E., Thornquist, M.D., Balmes, J., Cullen, M.R., Meyskens, F.L., Omenn, G.S., Valanis, B., & Williams, J.H. (2004). The beta-carotene and retinol efficacy trial: incidence of lung cancer and cardiovascular disease mortality during 6-year follow-up after stopping -carotene and retinol supplements. *Journal of the National Cancer Institute,* 96(23), 1743–1750.

104 Elles, M.P., Blaylock, M., & Huang, J. (2000). Plants as a natural source of concentrated mineral nutritional supplements. *Food Chemistry,* 71, 181–188.

105 Proevity Continuing Education Group. (2009). *How to evaluate vitamin and mineral products. What healthcare professionals want to know.* Retrieved from www.proevity cme.com

106 Ibid.

107 National Institute of Health. Office of Dietary Supplements. (2011). *Dietary supplements: background information*. Retrieved from http://ods.od.nih.gov/factsheets/dietarysup plements/

108 Cani, P.D., Delzenne, N.M., Amar, J., & Burcelin, R. (2008). Role of gut microflora in the development of obesity and insulin resistance following high-fat diet feeding. *Pathologie Biologie, 56,* 305–309.

109 Backhed, F., Ding, H., Wang, T., Hooper, L.V., Koh, G.Y., Nagy, A., Semenkovich, C.F., & Gordon, J.I. (2004). The gut microbiota as an environmental factor that regulates fat storage. *Proceedings of the National Academy of Sciences of the United States of America,* 101(44), 15718–15723.

110 Glycemic Index. (2011). *About glycemic index*. Retrieved from http://www.glycemicin dex.com/

111 National Institutes of Health. National Institute of Diabetes and Digestive and Kidney Disease. National Diabetes Information Clearinghouse. (2011). *Hypoglycemia*. Retrieved from http://diabetes.niddk.nih.gov/dm/pubs/hypoglycemia/#prevention

112 Glycemic Index. (2011). *About glycemic index*. Retrieved from http://www.glycemicin dex.com/

113 Johnson, R.K., Appel, L.J., Brands, M., Howard, B.V., Lefevre, M., Lustig, R.H., Sacks, F., Steffen, L.M., & Wylie-Rosett, J. (2009). Dietary sugars intake and cardiovascular health. A scientific statement from the American Heart Association. *Journal of the American Heart Association*. Retrieved from http://circ.ahajournals.org/content/120/11/1011.full.pdf+html

114 Ibid.

115 Ibid.

116 Avena, N.M., Rada, P., & Hoebel, B.G. (2007). Evidence for sugar addiction: behavioral and neurochemical effects of intermittent, excessive sugar intake. *Neuroscience and Biobehavioral Reviews,* 32(1), 20–39.

117 Parker, H. (2010). *A sweet problem: Princeton researchers find that high-fructose corn syrup prompts considerably more weight gain*. News at Princeton. Retrieved from http://www.princeton.edu/main/news/archive/S26/91/22K07/

118 Ibid.

119 Ibid.

120 Ibid.

121 Ibid.

122 Stanhope, K.L., & Havel, P.J. (2008). Endocrine and metabolic effects of consuming beverages sweetened with fructose, glucose, sucrose, or high-fructose corn syrup. *American Journal of Clinical Nutrition,* 88(6l), 1733S–1737S.

123 Norris, J. (2009). *Sugar is a poison, says UCSF obesity expert*. Retrieved from http://www.ucsf.edu/news/2009/06/8187/obesity-and-metabolic-syndrome-driven-fructose-sugar-diet

124 Ibid.

125 Weyand, C.M., & Goronzy, J.J. (1992). Clinically silent infections in patients with oligoarthritis: results of a prospective study. *Annals of Rheumatic Diseases,* 51(2), 253–258.

126 Fendler, C., Laitko, S., Sörensen, H., Gripenberg-Lerche, C., Groh, A., Uksila, J., Granfors, K., Braun, J., & Sieper, J. (2001). Frequency of triggering bacteria in patients with reactive arthritis and undifferentiated oligoarthritis and the relative importance of the tests used for diagnosis. *Annals of Rheumatic Disease*, 60(4), 337–343.

127 Bull, T.J., McMinn, E.J., Sidi-Boumedine, K., Skull, A., Durkin, D., Neild, P., Rhodes, G., Pickup, R., & Hermon-Taylor, J. (2003). Detection and verification of Mycobacterium avium subsp. paratuberculosis in fresh ileocolonic mucosal biopsy specimens from individuals with and without Crohn's disease. *Journal of Clinical Microbiology*, 41(7), 2915–2923.

128 Buzi, F., Badolato, R., Mazza, C., Giliani, S., Notarangelo, L.S., Radetti, G., Plebamo, A., & Notarangelo, L.D. (2003). Autoimmune polyendocrinopathy-Candidiasis-ectodermal dystrophy syndrome: time to review diagnostic criteria? *The Journal of Clinical Endocrinology & Metabolism*, 88(7), 3146–3148.

129 Vasquez, A. (2006). Reducing pain and inflammation naturally. Part 6: nutritional and botanical treatments against "silent infections" and gastrointestinal dysbiosis, commonly overlooked causes of neuromusculoskeletal inflammation and chronic health problems. Nutritional Perspectives. *Journal of the Council on Nutrition of the American Chiropractic Association*, 29(1), 5–21. Retrieved from: http://optimalhealthresearch.com/reprints/ series/ vasquez_part6_ 2006_dysbiosis

130 Backhed, F., Ding, H., Wang, T., Hooper, L.V., Koh, G.Y., Nagy, A., Semenkovich, C.F., & Gordon, J.I. (2004). The gut microbiota as an environmental factor that regulates fat storage. *Proceedings of the National Academy of Sciences of the United States of America*, 101(44), 15718–15723.

131 Babic, M., & Hukic, M. (2010). Candida albicans and non-albicans species as etiological agent of vaginitis in pregnant and non-pregnant women. *Bosnian Journal of Basic Medical Sciences*, 10(1), 89–97.

132 U.S. National Library of Medicine. National Institutes of Health. Medline Plus. (2010). *Seborrheic dermatiti*. Retrieved from http://www.nlm.nih.gov/medlineplus/ency/article/ 000963.htm

133 Brinkert, F., Sornsakrin, M., Krebs-Schmitt, D., & Ganschow, R. (2009). Chronic mucocutaneous candidiasis may cause elevated gliadin antibodies. *Acta Paediatrica*, 98(10), 1685–1688.

134 Shirtliff, M.E., Krom, B.P., Meijering, R. A., Peters, B.M., Zhu, J., Scheper, M.A., Harris, M.L., & Jabra-Rizk, M.A. (2009). Farnesol-induced apoptosis in Candida albicans. *Antimicrobrobial Agents and Chemotherapy*, 53(6), 2392–2401.

135 Merck. The Merck Manuals Online Medical Library. (2008). *Antibiotics*. Retrieved from http://www.merckmanuals.com/ home/sec17/ch192/ch192a.html?qt=antibiotics &alt=sh#sec17-ch192-ch192a-422

136 Merck. The Merck Manuals Online Medical Library. (2008). *Yeast infection (Candidiasis)*. Retrieved from http://www.merckmanuals.com/home/sec22/ch247/ ch247d.html?qt=yeast infection pregnancy&alt=sh

137 Merck. The Merck Manuals Online Medical Library. (2008). *Fungal infections introduction*. Retrieved from http://www.merckmanuals.com/home/sec17/ch197/ ch197a.html?qt=fungal%20infections%20infection&alt=sh

138 Guarro, J., Gené, J., & Stchigel, A.M. (1999). Developments in Fungal Taxonomy. *Clinical Microbiology Reviews*, 12(3) 454–500.

139 Ibid.

140 **Ibid.**

141 Galland, L. (1995). Leaky gut syndrome: breaking the vicious cycle, *Townsend Letter for Doctors*, 145(6), 63–68.

142 Kiefer, D., & Ali-Akbarian, L. (2004). A brief evidence-based review of two gastrointestinal illnesses: irritable bowel and leaky gut syndromes. *Alternative Therapies in Health and Medicine*, 10(3), 22–30.

143 Jackson, J.A., Riordan, H.D., Hunninghake, R., & Revard, C. (1999). Candida albicans: The hidden infection. *Journal of Orthomolecular Medicine*, 14(4), 198–200.

144 MDGuidelines (Medical Disability Guidelines). (2010). *Candidiasis*. Retrieved from http://www.mdguidelines.com/candidiasis/definition

145 Merck. The Merck Manuals Online Medical Library. (2008). *Fungal infections introduction*. Retrieved from http://www.merckmanuals.com/home/sec17/ch197/ch197a.html?qt=fungal%20infections%20infection&alt=sh

146 Rodaki, A., Bohovych, I.M., Enjalbert, B., Young, T., Odds, F.C., Gow, N.A., & Brown, A.J. (2009). Glucose promotes stress resistance in the fungal pathogen Candida albicans. *Source Molecular Biology of the Cell*, 20(22), 4845–4855.

147 Manns, J.M., Mosser, D.M., & Buckley, H.R. (1994). Production of a hemolytic factor by Candida albicans. *Infection and Immunity*, 62(11), 5154–5156.

148 Vasquez, A. (2006). Reducing pain and inflammation naturally. Part 6: nutritional and botanical treatments against "silent infections" and gastrointestinal dysbiosis, commonly overlooked causes of neuromusculoskeletal inflammation and chronic health problems. Nutritional Perspectives. *Journal of the Council on Nutrition of the American Chiropractic Association*, 29(1), 5–21. Retrieved from: http://optimalhealthresearch.com/reprints/series/ vasquez_part6_ 2006_dysbiosis

149 Galiatsatos, P., Gologan, A., & Lamoureux, E. (2009). Autistic enterocolitis: fact or fiction? *Canadian Journal of Gastroenterology*, 23(2), 95–98.

150 Vasquez, A. (2006). Reducing pain and inflammation naturally. Part 6: nutritional and botanical treatments against "silent infections" and gastrointestinal dysbiosis, commonly overlooked causes of neuromusculoskeletal inflammation and chronic health problems. Nutritional Perspectives. *Journal of the Council on Nutrition of the American Chiropractic Association*, 29(1), 5–21. Retrieved from: http://optimalhealthresearch.com/reprints/series/ vasquez_part6_ 2006_dysbiosis

151 Moraes, P.S. (1998). Recurrent vaginal candidiasis and allergic rhinitis: a common association. *Annals of Allergy, Asthma & Immunology*, 81(2), 165–169.

152 Neves, N.A., Carvalho, L.P., De Oliveira, M.A.M., Giraldo, P.C., Bacellar, O.,Cruz, A.A., & Carvalho, E.M. (2005). Association between atopy and recurrent vaginal candidiasis. *Clinical Experimental Immunology*, 142(1), 167–171.

153 National Institutes of Health. National Library of Medicine. National Center for Biotechnology Information. MedlinePlus. (2010). *Celiac disease—sprue*. Retrieved from http://www.ncbi.nlm.nih.gov/pubmedhealth/PMH0001280

154 Green, P., & Lebwohl, B. (2011). Mesalamine for refractory celiac disease: an old medicine for a new disease. *Journal of Clinical Gastroenterology*, 45(1), 1–3. Retrieved from http://journals.lww.com/jcge/Fulltext/2011/01000/Mesalamine_ for_ Refractory_Celiac_Disease__An_Old.1.aspx#

155 Martin, J.M., & Rona, Z. (1996). *Complete Candida yeast guidebook*. Rocklin, Ca: Prima Publishing.

156 Nieuwenhuizen, W.F., Pieters, R.H., Knippels, L.M., Jansen, M.C., & Koppelman, S.J. (2003). Is Candida albicans a trigger in the onset of coeliac disease? *Lancet*, 361(9375), 2152–2154.

157 Ibid.

158 Ibid.

159 Tursi, A., Brandimarte, G., & Giorgetti, G. (2003). High prevalence of small intestinal bacterial overgrowth in celiac patients with persistence of gastrointestinal symptoms after gluten withdrawal. *American Journal of Gastroenterology*, 98(4), 839–843.

160 Ibid.

161 Almeida, R.S., Wilson, D., & Hube, B. (2009). Candida albicans iron acquisition within the host. *FEMS Yeast Research*, 9(7), 1000–1012.

162 St Leger, R.J., Nelson, J.O., & Screen, S.E. (1999). The entomopathogenic fungus Metarhizium anisopliae alters ambient pH, allowing extracellular protease production and activity. *Microbiology*, 145, 2691–2699.

163 Tsuboi, R., Matsuda, K., Ko, I.J., & Ogawa, H. (1989). Correlation between culture medium pH, extracellular proteinase activity, and cell growth of Candida albicans in insoluble stratum corneum-supplemented media. *Archives of Dermatological Research*, 281(5), 342–345.

164 Cohen, S. (2010). *Candida yeast can hurt you (Part 1)*. Received from http://dearpharmacist.com/?p=1346

165 Glycemic Index. (2011). *About glycemic index*. Retrieved from http://www.glycemicindex.com/

166 Bohn, T., Davidson, L., Walczyk, T., & Hurrell, R.F. (2004). Phytic acid added to white-wheat bread inhibits fractional apparent magnesium absorption in humans. *American Journal of Clinical Nutrition*, 79(3), 418–423.

167 Ibid.

168 Ibid.

169 Gilbert, S.G., Bellinger, D.C., Goldman, L.R., Grandjean, P., Herbert, M.R., Landrigan, P.J., Lanphear, B.P., McElgunn, B., Myers, J.P., Pessah, I., Schettler, T., & Weiss, B. (2010). *Scientific consensus statement on environmental agents associated with neuro-developmental disorders*. Collaborative on Health and the Environment's Learning and Developmental Disabilities Initiative. Retrieved from http://www.fluoridealert.org/scientific.consensus.nov.2007.pdf

170 PBS. (2010). *The problem. Trade secrets*. Reviewed from http://www.pbs.org/trade secrets/problem/problem.html

171 Nugent, S. (2004). *How to survive on a toxic planet*. US: Alethia Corporation.

172 Gilbert, S.G., Bellinger, D.C., Goldman, L.R., Grandjean, P., Herbert, M.R., Landrigan, P.J., Lanphear, B.P., McElgunn, B., Myers, J.P., Pessah, I., Schettler, T., & Weiss,. B. (2010). *Scientific consensus statement on environmental agents associated with neuro-developmental disorders*. Collaborative on Health and the Environment's Learning and Developmental Disabilities Initiative. Retrieved from http://www.fluoridealert.org/scientific.consensus.nov.2007.pdf

173 Ibid.

174 Nakazawa, D.J. (2008). *The autoimmune epidemic*. New York, NY: Touchstone.

175 Centers of Disease Control and Prevention. (2010). *National report on human exposure to environmental chemicals.* Received from http://www.cdc.gov/exposurereport/Gen eral_FactSheet.html

176 Gilbert, S.G., Bellinger, D.C., Goldman, L.R., Grandjean, P., Herbert, M.R., Landrigan, P.J., Lanphear, B.P., McElgunn, B., Myers, J.P., Pessah, I., Schettler, T., & Weiss,. B. (2010). *Scientific consensus statement on environmental agents associated with neuro-developmental disorders.* Collaborative on Health and the Environment's Learning and Developmental Disabilities Initiative. Retrieved from http://www.fluoridealert.org/ scientific.consensus.nov.2007.pdf

177 Ghali, N., & Josifova, D. (2010). Genetic investigations in children with learning difficulties. *Acta Neurobiologiae Experimentalis, 70,* 165–176.

178 Gilbert, S.G., Bellinger, D.C., Goldman, L.R., Grandjean, P., Herbert, M.R., Landrigan, P.J., Lanphear, B.P., McElgunn, B., Myers, J.P., Pessah, I., Schettler, T., & Weiss,. B. (2010). *Scientific consensus statement on environmental agents associated with neuro-developmental disorders.* Collaborative on Health and the Environment's Learning and Developmental Disabilities Initiative. Retrieved from http://www.fluoridealert.org/ scientific.consensus.nov.2007.pdf

179 Ibid.

180 Wallinga, D., Sorensen, J., Mottl, P., & Yablon, B. (2009). *Not so sweet: missing mercury and high fructose corn syrup.* Institute for Agriculture and Trade Policy. Retrieved from http://www.healthobservatory.org/library.cfm?refid=105026

181 National Cancer Institute. U.S. National Institutes of Health. (2010). *Cancer trends progress report—2009/2010 update.* Retrieved from http://progressreport.cancer.gov/ doc_detail.asp?pid=1&did=2009&chid=91&coid=906&mid=#trends

182 Ibid.

183 Ibid.

184 Rajapakse, N., Silva, E., and Kortenkamp, A. (2002). Combining xenoestrogens at levels below individual no-observed-effect concentrations dramatically enhances steroid hormone action. *Environmental Health Perspectives, 110*(9), 917–921. Retrieved from http://www.ncbi.nlm.nih.gov/pmc/articles/PMC1240992/pdf/ehp0110-000917.pdf

185 Costello, T. (2004). *Male fish becoming female.* NBC News. MSN. Received from http://www.msnbc.msn.com/id/6436617/

186 Jeffries, K.M., Jackson, L.J., Ikonomou, M.G., & Habib, H.R. (2010). Presence of natural and anthropogenic organic contaminants and potential fish health impacts along two river gradients in Alberta, Canada. *Environmental Toxicology and Chemistry, 29*(10), 2379–2387. doi: 10.1002/etc.265

187 Ibid.

188 Dearing, S. (2010). Chemicals turning male fish into female fish in Alberta rivers. *Digital Journal.* Retrieved from http://www.digitaljournal.com/article/295321

189 U.S. Environmental Protection Agency. (2011). *Table of products that may contain mercury and recommended management options.* Retrieved from http://www.epa.gov/ osw/hazard/tsd/mercury/con-prod.htm

190 U.S. Environmental Protection Agency. (2010). *Mercury. Basic information.* Retrieved from http://www.epa.gov/hg/about.htm

191 U.S. Environmental Protection Agency. (2011). *Mercury. Health effects.* Retrieved from http://www.epa.gov/mercury/effects.htm

192 U.S. Environmental Protection Agency. (2010). *Human exposure. Methylmercury exposure.* Retrieved from http://www.epa.gov/earlink1/mercury/exposure.htm

193 Ramirez, G.B., Pagulayan, O., Akagi, H., Francisco Rivera, A., Lee, L.V., Berroya, A., Vince Cruz, M.C., & Casintahan, D. (2003). Tagum study II: Follow-up study at two years of age after prenatal exposure to mercury. *Pediatrics*, 111(3), e289–295.

194 U.S. Environmental Protection Agency. (2010). *Human exposure. Methylmercury exposure.* Retrieved from http://www.epa.gov/earlink1/mercury/exposure.htm

195 CBC News. (2010). *FDA reopens debate on dental amalgam fillings.* Retrieved from http://www.cbc.ca/health/story/2010/06/11/con-amalgam-hearing.html

196 Björkman, L., Sandborgh-Englund, G., & Ekstrand, J. (1997). Mercury in saliva and feces after removal of amalgam fillings. *Toxicology and Applied Pharmacology*, 144(1), 156–162.

197 Stablum, A. (2007). *EU faces pressure to ban mercury from mouths.* Reuters. Retrieved from http://www.reuters.com/article/2007/07/25/us-mercury-eu-amalgams-idUSL2319134520070725?pageNumber=2

198 U.S. Environmental Protection Agency. (2010). *Dental amalgam effluent guideline.* Retrieved from http://water.epa.gov/scitech/wastetech/guide/dental/index.cfm

199 Ibid.

200 Ibid.

201 Luster, M., & Rosenthal, G.J. (1993). Chemical agents and the immune response. *Environmental Health Perspectives*, 100, 219–236.

202 Inadera, H. (2006). The immune system as a target for environmental chemicals: xenoestrogens and other compounds. *Toxicology Letters*, 164(3), 191–206.

203 Ibid.

204 Ibid.

205 Ibid.

206 Villeneuve, S., Cyr, D., Lynge, E., Orsi, L., Sabroe, S., Merletti, F., Gorini, G., Morales-Suarez-Varela, M., Ahrens, W., Baumgardt-Elms, C., Kaerlev, L., Eriksson, M., Hardell, L., Févotte, J., & Guénel, P. (2010). Occupation and occupational exposure to endocrine disrupting chemicals in male breast cancer: a case-control study in Europe. *Occupational and Environmental Medicine*, 12, 837–844.

207 Belpomme, D., Irigaray, P., Osspmdp, M., Vacque, D., & Martin, M. (2009). Prostate cancer as an environmental disease: an ecological study in the French Caribbean islands, Martinique and Guadeloupe. *International Journal of Oncology*, 34, 1037–1044.

208 Gouveia-Vigeant, T., & Tickner, J. (2003). *Toxic chemicals and childhood cancer: a review of the evidence.* Retrieved from http://www.sustainableproduction.org/downloads/Child%20Canc%20Exec%20Summary.pdf

209 Bouchard, M.F., Bellinger, D.C., Wright, R.O., & Weisskopf, M.G. (2010). Attention-deficit/hyperactivity disorder and urinary metabolites of organophosphate pesticides. *Pediatrics*, doi: 10.1542/peds.2009–3058. Retrieved from http://pediatrics.aappublications.org/content/early/2010/05/17/peds.2009-3058.full.pdf+html

210 Morgan, D.L., Chanda, S.M., Price, H.C., Fernando, R., Liu, L., Brambila, E., O'Connor, R.W., Beliles, R.P., & Barone, S. (2002). Disposition of inhaled mercury vapor in pregnant rats: maternal toxicity and effects on developmental outcome. *Toxicological Sciences*, 66(2), 261–273.

211 Ramirez, G.B., Pagulayan, O., Akagi, H., Francisco Rivera, A., Lee, L.V., Berroya, A., Vince Cruz, M.C., & Casintahan, D. (2003). Tagum study II: follow-up study at two years of age after prenatal exposure to mercury. *Pediatrics*, 111(3), e289–295.

212 U.S. Environmental Protection Agency. (2010). *Human exposure. Methylmercury exposure*. Retrieved from http://www.epa.gov/earlink1/mercury/exposure.htm

213 Kogan, M.D., Blumberg, S.J., Schieve, L.A., Boyle, C.A., Perrin, J.M., Ghandour, R.M., Singh, G.K., Strickland, B.B., Trevathan, E., & Van Dyck, P.C. (2009). Prevalence of parent-reported diagnosis of autism spectrum disorder among children in the U.S., 2007. *Pediatrics*, 124(5), 1395–1403. doi:10.1542/peds.2009–1522

214 Kennedy, R. (2005). *Tobacco science and the thimerosal scandal*. Retrieved from http://www.robertfkennedyjr.com/docs/ThimerosalScandalFINAL.PDF

215 Ibid.

216 U.S. Department of Health and Human Services. U.S. Food and Drug Administration. (2010). *Thimerosal in vaccines*. Retrieved from http://www.fda.gov/BiologicsBloodVac cines/SafetyAvailability/VaccineSafety/UCM096228

217 DeSoto, M.C., & Hitlan, R.T. (2010). Sorting out the spinning of autism: heavy metals and the question of incidence. *Acta Neurobiologiae Experimentalis*, 70, 165–176.

218 Vasquez, A. (2006). Reducing pain and inflammation naturally. Part 6: nutritional and botanical treatments against "silent infections" and gastrointestinal dysbiosis, commonly overlooked causes of neuromusculoskeletal inflammation and chronic health problems. Nutritional Perspectives. *Journal of the Council on Nutrition of the American Chiropractic Association*, 29(1), 5–21. Retrieved from: http://optimalhealthresearch.com/reprints/ series/ vasquez_part6_ 2006_dysbiosis

219 Ibid.

220 Biotics Research Corporation. (2011). *Announcing Dr. Alex Vasquez as the Director of the Medical Board of Advisors for Biotics Research Corporation*. Retrieved from http://www.bioticsresearch.com/node/2434

221 Vasquez, A. (2006). Reducing pain and inflammation naturally. Part 6: nutritional and botanical treatments against "silent infections" and gastrointestinal dysbiosis, commonly overlooked causes of neuromusculoskeletal inflammation and chronic health problems. Nutritional Perspectives. *Journal of the Council on Nutrition of the American Chiropractic Association*, 29(1), 5–21. Retrieved from: http://optimalhealthresearch.com/reprints/ series/ vasquez_part6_ 2006_dysbiosis

222 Dean, C. (2008). *Depression and yeast*. Doctor of the Future Publications. Retrieved from http://drcarolyndean.com/articles_depression_and_yeast.html

223 Ogasawara, O., Odahara, K., Toume, M., Watanabe, T., Mikami, T., & Matsumoto, T. (2006). Change in the respiration system of Candida albicans in the lag and log growth phase. *Biological and Pharmaceutical Bulletin*, 29(3), 448–450.

224 Spinucci, G., Guidetti, M., Lanzoni, E., & Pironi, L. (2006). Endogenous ethanol production in a patient with chronic intestinal pseudo-obstruction and small intestinal bacterial overgrowth. European Journal of Gastroenterology & Hepatology, 18(7), 799–802.

225 Kurkivuori, J., Salaspuro, V., Kaihovaara, P., Kari, K., Rautemaa, R., Grönroos, L., Meurman, J.H., & Salaspuro, M. (2007). Acetaldehyde production from ethanol by oral streptococci. Oral Oncology, 43(2), 181–186.

226 Spinucci, G., Guidetti, M., Lanzoni, E., & Pironi, L. (2006). Endogenous ethanol production in a patient with chronic intestinal pseudo-obstruction and small intestinal bacterial overgrowth. *European Journal of Gastroenterology & Hepatology*, 18(7), 799–802.

227 Kaminishi, H., Miyaguchi, H., Tamaki, T., Suenaga, N., Hisamatsu, M., Mihashi, I., Matsumoto, H., Maeda, H., & Hagihara, Y. (1995). Degradation of humoral host defense by Candida albicans proteinase. *Infection and Immununity*, 63(3), 984–988.

228 Douglas, L.J. (1988). Candida proteinases and candidosis. *Critical Reviews in Biotechnology*, 8(2), 121–129.

229 Vasquez, A. (2006). Reducing pain and inflammation naturally. Part 6: nutritional and botanical treatments against "silent infections" and gastrointestinal dysbiosis, commonly overlooked causes of neuromusculoskeletal inflammation and chronic health problems. Nutritional Perspectives. *Journal of the Council on Nutrition of the American Chiropractic Association*, 29(1), 5–21. Retrieved from: http://optimalhealthresearch.com/reprints/series/vasquez_part6_2006_dysbiosis

230 Douglas, L.J. (1988). Candida proteinases and candidosis. *Critical Reviews in Biotechnology*, 8(2), 121–129.

231 Sutton, P., Newcombe, N.R., Waring, P., & Mullbacher, A. (1994). In vivo immunosuppressive activity of gliotoxin, a metabolite produced by human pathogenic fungi. *Infection and Immunity*, 62(4), 1192–1198.

232 Shah, D.T., Glover, D.D., Larsen, B. (1995). In situ mycotoxin production by Candida albicans in women with vaginitis. *Gynecologic and Obstetric Investigation*, 39, 67–69.

233 Shah, D.T., Larsen, B. (1991). Clinical isolates of yeast produce a gliotoxin-like substance. *Mycopathologia*, 116, 203–208.

234 Waring, P., & Beaver, J. (1996). Gliotoxin and related epipolythiodioxopiperazines. *General Pharmacology*, 27, 1311–1316.

235 Kaji, H., Asanuma, Y., Yahara, O., Shibue, H., Hisamura, M., Saito, N., Kawakami, Y., & Murao, M. (1984). Intragastrointestinal alcohol fermentation syndrome: report of two cases and review of the literature. *Journal of the Forensic Science Society*, 24(5), 461–471.

236 Jansson-Nettelbladt, E., Meurling, S., Petrini, B., & Sjölin, J. (1995). Endogenous ethanol fermentation in a child with short bowel syndrome. *Acta Paediatrica*, 95(4), 502–504.

237 Kurkivuori, J., Salaspuro, V., Kaihovaara, P., Kari, K., Rautemaa, R., Grönroos, L., Meurman, J.H., & Salaspuro, M. (2007). Acetaldehyde production from ethanol by oral streptococci. *Oral Oncology*, 43(2), 181–186.

238 Mukherjee, P.K., Mohamed, S., Chandra, J., Kuhn, D., Liu, S., Antar, O.S., Munyon, R., Mitchell, A.P., Andes, D., Chance, M., Rouabhia, M., & Ghannoum, M.A. (2006). Alcohol dehydrogenase restricts the ability of the pathogen Candida albicans to form a biofilm on catheter surfaces through an ethanol-based mechanism. *Infection and Immunity*, 74(7), 3804–3816.

239 Ghosh, S., Kebaara, B.W., Atkin, A.L., & Nickerson, K.W. (2008). Regulation of aromatic alcohol production in Candida albicans. *Applied and Environmental Microbiology*, 74(23), 7211–7218.

240 Ibid

241 Kosalec, I., Safrani, A., Pepeljnjak, S., Bacun-Druzina, V., Rami, S., & Kopjar, N. (2008). Genotoxicity of tryptophol in a battery of short-term assays on human white blood cells in vitro. *Basic & Clinical Pharmacology & Toxicology*, 102(5), 443–452.

242 Kaminishi, H., Miyaguchi, H., Tamaki, T., Suenaga, N., Hisamatsu, M., Mihashi, I., Matsumoto, H., Maeda, H., & Hagihara, Y. (1995). Degradation of humoral host defense by Candida albicans proteinase. *Infection and Immununity*, 63(3), 984–988.

243 Douglas, L.J. (1988). Candida proteinases and candidosis. *Critical Reviews in Biotechnology*, 8(2), 121–129.

244 Great Plains Laboratory Inc. (2011). *Clinical significance of the Organic Acids Test. General indicators of gastrointestinal dysbiosis.* Retrieved from http://www.greatplains laboratory.com/home/eng/Clinical%20Significance%20of%20the%20OAT.pdf

245 Noverr, M.C., Toews, G.B., & Huffnagle, G.B. (2002). Production of prostaglandins and leukotrienes by pathogenic fungi. *Infection and Immunity*, 70(1), 400–402. doi: 10.1128/IAI.70.1.400–402.2002

246 Noverr, M.C., Phare, S.M., Toews, G.B., Coffey, M.J., & Huffnagle, G.B. (2001). Pathogenic yeasts Cryptococcus neoformans and Candida albicans produce immunomodulatory prostaglandins. *Infection and Immunity*, 69(5), 2957–2963.

247 Sakai, Y., & Tani, Y. (1987). Formaldehyde production with heat-treated cells of methanol yeast. *Journal of Fermentation Technology*, 65(4), 489–491.

248 Noverr, M.C., Toews, G.B., & Huffnagle, G.B. (2002). Production of prostaglandins and leukotrienes by pathogenic fungi. *Infection and Immunity*, 70(1), 400–402. doi: 10.1128/IAI.70.1.400–402.2002

249 Branum, A.M., & Lukacs, S.L. (2008). *Food allergy among U.S. children: trends in prevalence and hospitalizations.* NCH Data brief, 10. U.S. Department of Health and Human Services. Centers for Disease Control and Prevention. National Center for Health Statistics. Retrieved from http://www.cdc.gov/nchs/data/databriefs/db10.pdf

250 American Academy of Allergy and Asthma and Immunology. (2011). *Allergy statistics.* Retrieved from http://www.aaaai.org/media/statistics/allergy-statistics.asp

251 CBC News. (2010). *Seasonal allergies: something to sneeze at.* Retrieved from http://www.cbc.ca/news/health/story/2010/03/19/f-seasonal-allergies-symptoms.html

252 Branum, A.M., & Lukacs, S.L. (2008). *Food allergy among U.S. children: trends in prevalence and hospitalizations.* NCH Data brief, 10. U.S. Department of Health and Human Services. Centers for Disease Control and Prevention. National Center for Health Statistics. Retrieved from http://www.cdc.gov/nchs/data/databriefs/db10.pdf

253 Ibid.

254 Noverr, M.C., Toews, G.B., & Huffnagle, G.B. (2002). Production of prostaglandins and leukotrienes by pathogenic fungi. *Infection and Immunity*, 70(1), 400–402. doi: 10.1128/IAI.70.1.400–402.2002

255 Ponikau, J.U., Sherris, D.A., Kern, E.B., Homburger, H.A., Frigas, E., Gaffey, T.A., & Roberts, G.D. (2009). The diagnosis and incidence of allergic fungal sinusitis. *Mayo Clinic Proceedings*, 74(9), 877–884.

256 Ibid.

257 Noverr, M.C., Toews, G.B., & Huffnagle, G.B. (2002). Production of prostaglandins and leukotrienes by pathogenic fungi. *Infection and Immunity*, 70(1), 400–402. doi: 10.1128/IAI.70.1.400–402.2002

258 Asthma Society of Canada. (2011). *Treatment. All about inhaled steroids.* Retrieved from http://www.asthma.ca/adults/treatment/steroids.php

259 Ibid.

260 French, T.W., Blue, J.T., & Stokol, T. (2011). *Clinical blood glucose, carbohydrates and lipids*. Chemistry basics. eClinPath. Cornell University College of Veterinary Medicine. Retrieved from http://ahdc.vet.cornell.edu/clinpath/modules/chem/GLUCOSE.HTM

261 Vasquez, A. (2006). Reducing pain and inflammation naturally. Part 6: nutritional and botanical treatments against "silent infections" and gastrointestinal dysbiosis, commonly overlooked causes of neuromusculoskeletal inflammation and chronic health problems. Nutritional Perspectives. *Journal of the Council on Nutrition of the American Chiropractic Association*, 29(1), 5–21. Retrieved from: http://optimalheal thresearch.com/reprints/series/ vasquez_part6_ 2006_dysbiosis

262 Patlak, M. (2005). *Your guide to healthy sleep*. U.S. Department of health and Human Services, National Institutes of Health, National Heart, Lung, and Blood Institute. Retrieved from http://www.nhlbi.nih.gov/health/public/sleep/healthy_sleep.pdf

263 Ibid.

264 Ibid.

265 Ibid.

266 Mayo Clinic. (2009). *Exercise: 7 benefits of regular physical activity*. Retrieved from http://www.mayoclinic.com/health/exercise/HQ01676/METHOD=print

267 American College of Sports Medicine (ACSM). (2010). *Physical activities and health guidelines*. Retrieved from http://www.acsm.org/AM/Template.cfm?Section=Home_ Page&TEMPLATE=CM/HTMLDisplay.cfm&CONTENTID=7764#Tips_For_Meet ing_Guidelines

268 American Heart Association. (2011). *American Heart Association guidelines. Physical activity*. Retrieved from http://www.heart.org/HEARTORG/GettingHealthy/ PhysicalActivity/GettingActive/American-Heart-Association-Guidelines_ UCM_307976_Article.jsp

269 Smedby, K.E., Hjalgrim, H., Melbye, M., Torrång, A., Rostgaard, K., Munksgaard, L., Adami, J., Hansen, M., Porwit-MacDonald, A., Jensen, B.A., Roos, G., Pedersen, B.B., Sundström, C., Glimelius, B., & Adami, H.O. (2005). Ultraviolet radiation exposure and risk of malignant lymphomas. *Journal of the National Cancer Institute*, 97, 199–209. doi: 0.1093/jnci/dji022

270 Berwick, M., Armstrong, B.K., Ben-Porat, L., Fine, J., Kricker, A., & Eberle, C. (2005). Sun exposure and mortality from melanoma. *The National Cancer Institute*, 97, 195–199.

271 Mead, M.N. (2008). Benefits of sunlight a bright spot for human health. *Environmental Health Perspectives*, 116(4), A161–167. Retrieved from http://ehp.niehs.nih.gov/mem bers/2008/116–4/EHP116pa160PDF

272 Ibid.

273 McMichael, A.J., Lucas, R., Ponsonby, A.L., & Edwards, S.J. (2009). Chapter 8. Stratospheric ozone depletion, ultraviolet radiation and health. *Climate Change and Human Health*. World Health Organization. (pp 159–180). Retrieved from http:// www.who.int/globalchange/publications/climatechangechap8.pdf

274 Mead, M.N. (2008). Benefits of sunlight a bright spot for human health. *Environmental Health Perspectives*, 116(4), A161–167. Retrieved from http://ehp.niehs.nih.gov/mem bers/2008/116-4/EHP116pa160PDF

SECTION THREE

275 Mathur, S., Mathur, R.S., Dowda, H., Williamson, H.O., Faulk, W.P., & Fudenberg, H.H. (1978). Sex hormones and antibodies to Candida albicans. *Clinical and Experimental Immunology*, 33(1), 79–87.

276 Livingstone, C., & Collison, M. (2002). Sex steroids and insulin resistance. *Clinical Science*, 102, 151–166.

277 Ahmed, S.A., Penhale, W.J., & Talal, N. (1985). Sex hormones, immune responses, and autoimmune diseases. Mechanisms of sex hormone action. *American Journal of Pathology*, 121(3), 531–551.

278 Miguel, J., Pulido, E., & Salazar, M.A. (1999). Changes in insulin sensitivity, secretion and glucose effectiveness during menstrual cycle. *Archives of Medical Research*, 30, 19–22.

279 Moore, J., Barlow, D., Jewell, D., & Kennedy, S. (1998). Do gastrointestinal symptoms vary with the menstrual cycle? *British Journal of Obstetrics and Gynaecology*, 105(12), 1322–1325.

280 Critchley, H.O.D., Kelly, R.W., Brenner, R.M., & Baird, D.T. (2001). The endocrinology of menstruation—a role for the immune system. *Clinical Endocrinology*, 55, 701–710.

281 Ibid.

282 Noverr, M.C., Toews, G.B. & Huffnagle, G.B. (2002). Production of prostaglandins and leukotrienes by pathogenic fungi. *Infection and Immunity*, 70(1), 400–402. doi: 10.1128/IAI.70.1.400–402.2002

283 U.S. Department of Health and Human Services. Woman's Health. (2010). *Premenstrual syndrome*. Retrieved from http://www.womenshealth.gov/faq/premenstrual-syndrome.cfm

284 Vasquez, A. (2006). Reducing pain and inflammation naturally. Part 6: nutritional and botanical treatments against "silent infections" and gastrointestinal dysbiosis, commonly overlooked causes of neuromusculoskeletal inflammation and chronic health problems. Nutritional Perspectives. *Journal of the Council on Nutrition of the American Chiropractic Association*, 29(1), 5–21. Retrieved from: http://optimalhealthresearch.com/reprints/series/ vasquez_part6_ 2006_dysbiosis

285 Sutton, P., Newcombe, N.R., Waring, P. & Mullbacher, A. (1994). In vivo immuno-suppressive activity of gliotoxin, a metabolite produced by human pathogenic fungi. *Infection and Immunity*, 62(4), 1192–1198.

286 Vasquez, A. (2006). Reducing pain and inflammation naturally. Part 6: nutritional and botanical treatments against "silent infections" and gastrointestinal dysbiosis, commonly overlooked causes of neuromusculoskeletal inflammation and chronic health problems. Nutritional Perspectives. *Journal of the Council on Nutrition of the American Chiropractic Association*, 29(1), 5–21. Retrieved from: http://optimalhealthresearch.com/reprints/series/ vasquez_part6_ 2006_dysbiosis

287 Moraes, P., Santos, F., Horizonte, B. (1998). Recurrent vaginal candidiasis and allergic rhinitis: a common association. *Annals of Allergy Asthma and Immunology*, 2, 165–169.

288 Miles, M.R., Olsen, L., & Rogers, A. (1977). Recurrent vaginal candidiasis. Importance of an intestinal reservoir. *Journal of the American Medical Association*, 238(17), 1836–1837.

289 Merck. The Merck Manuals Online Medical Library. (2008). *Yeast infection (Candidiasis)*. Retrieved from http://www.merckmanuals.com/home/sec22/ch247/ch247d html?qt=yeast infection pregnancy&alt=sh

290 National Institute of Health. (2011). *Assessment of alterations in immune function during pregnancy and post parturition.* Retrieved from http://clinicaltrials.gov/ct2/show/NCT01200979

291 Ibid.

292 McCracken, S.A., Gallery, E., & Morris, J.M. (2004). Pregnancy-specific down-regulation of NF-KB expression in T cells in humans is essential for the maintenance of the cytokine profile required for pregnancy success. *Journal of Immunology, 172,* 4583–4591.

293 Guerin, L.R., Prins, J.R., Robertson, S.A. (2009). Regulatory T-cells and immune tolerance in pregnancy: a new target for infertility treatment? *Human Reproduction Update,* 15(5), 517–535.

294 Moore, A.G., Brown, D.A., Fairlie, W.D., Bauskin, A.R., Brown, P.K., Munier, M.L.C., Russel, P.K., Salamonsen, L.A., Wallace, E.M., & Breit, S.N. (2000). The transforming growth factor-β superfamily cytokine macrophage inhibitory cytokine—1 is present in high concentrations in the serum of pregnant women. *Journal of Clinical Endocrinology and Metabolism,* 85, 4781–4788.

295 Butte, N. (2000). Carbohydrate and lipid metabolism in pregnancy: normal compared with gestational diabetes mellitus. *American Journal of Clinical Nutrition,* 71(5), 1256S–1261S.

296 Ibid.

297 Gonçalves, L.F., Chaiworapongsa, T., & Romero, R. (2002). Intrauterine infection and prematurity. *Mental Retardation Developmental Disabilities,* 8(1), 3–13.

298 Monga, M., Blanco, J.D. (1995). Intrauterine Infection and Preterm Labor. *Infectious Diseases in Obstetrics and Gynecology,* 3(1), 37–44.

299 Ibid.

300 Ibid.

301 Ibid

302 U.S. Department of Health and Human Services. National Institute of Health. MedlinePlus. (2011). *Iron in diet.* Retrieved from http://www.nlm.nih.gov/medlineplus/ency/article/002422.htm

303 U.S. Department of Health and Human Services. National Institute of Health. MedlinePlus. (2011). *Menstrual periods—heavy, prolonged, or irregular.* Retrieved from http://www.nlm.nih.gov/medlineplus/ency/article/003263.htm

304 U.S. Department of Health and Human Services. National Institute of Health. National Institute of Diabetes and Digestive and Kidney Disease. National Hematologic Diseases Information Service. (2011). *Anemia of inflammation and chronic disease.* Retrieved from http://hematologic.niddk.nih.gov/anemiachronic.aspx

305 Ibid.

306 Almeida, R.S., Wilson, D., & Hube, B. (2009). Candida albicans iron acquisition within the host. *FEMS Yeast Research,* 9(7), 1000–1012.

307 Garcia, Y.H., Díez, S.G., Aizpún, L.T., & Oliva, N.P. (2002). Antigliadin antibodies associated with chronic mucocutaneous Candidiasis. *Pediatric Dermatology,* 19(5), 415–418.

308 Brinkert, F., Sornsakrin, M., Krebs-Schmitt, D., & Ganschow, R. (2009). Chronic mucocutaneous candidiasis may cause elevated gliadin antibodies. *Acta Paediatrica,* 98(10), 1685–1688.

309 Garcia, Y.H., Díez, S.G., Aizpún, L.T., & Oliva, N.P. (2002). Antigliadin antibodies associated with chronic mucocutaneous Candidiasis. *Pediatric Dermatology*, 19(5), 415–418.

310 Ibid.

311 Brinkert, F., Sornsakrin, M., Krebs-Schmitt, D., & Ganschow, R. (2009). Chronic mucocutaneous candidiasis may cause elevated gliadin antibodies. *Acta Paediatrica*, 98(10), 1685–1688.

312 U.S. Department of Health and Human Services. Woman's Health. (2009). *Endometriosis*. Retrieved from http://www.womenshealth.gov/faq/endometriosis.cfm#a

313 National Institutes of Health. (2009). *Endometriosis*. Retrieved from http://www.ncbi.nlm.nih.gov/pubmedhealth/PMH0001913

314 U.S. Department of Health and Human Services. Woman's Health. (2009). *Endometriosis*. Retrieved from http://www.womenshealth.gov/faq/endometriosis.cfm#a

315 Luscombe, G., Markham, R., Judio, M., Grigoriu, A., & Fraser, I. (2009). Abdominal bloating: an under-recognized endometriosis symptom. *Journal of Obstetrics and Gynecology Canada*, 12, 1159–1171.

316 Sinaii, N., Cleary, S., Ballweg, M., Nieman, L., & Stratton, P. (2002). High rates of autoimmune and endocrine disorders, fibromyalgia, chronic fatigue syndrome and atopic diseases among women with endometriosis: a survey analysis. *Human Reproduction*, 17(10), 2715–2724.

317 U.S. Department of Health and Human Services. Woman's Health. (2009). *Endometriosis*. Retrieved from http://www.womenshealth.gov/faq/endometriosis.cfm#a

318 Antonelli, A., Campatelli, A., Di Vito, A., Alberti, B., Baldi, V., Salvioni, G., Fallahi, P., & Baschieri, L. (1994). Comparison between ethanol sclerotherapy and emptying with injection of saline in treatment of thyroid cysts. *Clinical Investigator*, 72(12), 971–974.

319 Ibid.

320 Simoncini, T. (2007). Cancer is a fungus. *A revolution in tumor therapy*. Italy: Edizioni Lampis.

321 Canadian Center for Occupational Health and Safety. (2005). *What is an LD50 and LC50?* Government of Canada. Retrieved from http://www.ccohs.ca/oshanswers/chemicals/ld50.html#_1_1

322 Santelli, J., Rochat, R., Hatfield-Timajchy, K., Colley Gilbert, B., Curtis, K., Cabral, R., Hirsch, J.S., & Schieve, L. (2003). The measurement and meaning of unintended pregnancy. *Perspectives on Sexual and Reproductive Health*, 35(2), 94–101.

323 Guttmacher Institute. (2011). *An Overview of Abortion in the United States*. Retrieved from http://www.guttmacher.org/presentations/abort_slides.pdf

324 Ibid.

325 Ibid.

326 Ibid.

327 Physician's Desk Reference. (2011). *Concise Monograph for Mifeprex*. Retrieved from http://www.pdr.net/drugpages/concisemonograph.aspx?concise=1759#warnings

328 CBC News. (2010). *Birth control users sue Bayer*. Retrieved from http://www.cbc.ca/health/story/2010/03/11/yasmin-yaz-birth-control-lawsuits-bayer.html

329 Physician's Desk Reference. (2011). *Concise Monograph for Yasmin*. Retrieved from http://www.pdr.net/drugpages/concisemonograph.aspx?concise=1758

330 Santelli, J., Rochat, R., Hatfield-Timajchy, K., Colley Gilbert, B., Curtis, K., Cabral, R., Hirsch, J.S., & Schieve, L. (2003). The measurement and meaning of unintended pregnancy. *Perspectives on Sexual and Reproductive Health*, 35(2), 94–101.

331 Wise, A., Brien, S., & Woodruff, T. (2011). Are oral contraceptives a significant contributor to the estrogenicity of drinking water? *Environmental Science & Technology*, 45, 51–60.

332 Ibid.

333 Wise, A., Brien, S., & Woodruff, T. (2011). Are oral contraceptives a significant contributor to the estrogenicity of drinking water? *Environmental Science & Technology*, 45, 51–60.

334 U.S. Department of Health and Human Services. Woman's Health. (2009). *Birth control methods*. Retrieved from http://www.womenshealth.gov/faq/birth-control-methods.pdf

335 American Pregnancy Association. (2011). *Overview: birth control*. Retrieved from http://www.americanpregnancy.org/preventingpregnancy/birthcontrolfailure.html

336 Mota, N.P., Burnett, M., Sareen, J. (2010). Associations between abortion, mental disorders and suicidal behavior in a nationally representative sample. *The Canadian Journal of Psychiatry*, 55(4), 239–247.

337 Coleman, P.K. (2009). *Does abortion cause mental health problems? The evidence through an objective scientific lens as opposed to the APA's recent analysis*. The American Association of Prolife Obstetrics and Gynaecologists. Retrieved from http://aaplog.octoberblue.com/wp-content/uploads/2010/02/Abortion-and-Mental-Health-Coleman-08.pdf

338 U.S. Department of Health and Human Services. Woman's Health. (2009). *Birth control methods*. Retrieved from http://www.womenshealth.gov/faq/birth-control-methods.pdf

339 Creighton Model. (2011). *Creighton Model. FertilityCare System*. Retrieved from http://www.creightonmodel.com/index.html

340 Fehring, R.J., Lawrence, D., & Philpot, C. (1994). Use effectiveness of the Creighton model ovulation method of natural family planning. *Journal of Obstetric, Gynaecologic, and Neonatal Nursing*, 23(4), 303–309.

SECTION FOUR

341 Morice, R. (2011). *About Ryan Morice. Adventure capital the 7 Summits*. Retrieved from http://adventurecapital7s.blogspot.com/p/about-ryan-morice.html

342 Ibid.

INDEX

Lightning Source UK Ltd.
Milton Keynes UK
UKHW021911171218
334165UK00026B/1507/P